The Grocery Store Myth

Copyright © 2008 by Eve Clark

All rights reserved. No part of this text may be reproduced by any means in any form whatsoever in electronic or mechanical, including photocopying, recording and information storage without written permission from the author, except for brief quotations embodied in literary article or reviews.

Disclaimer

This book is for informational purposes only. It is not intended to diagnose, prevent or treat any diseases. This is only a helpful guideline for healthy living.

Copyright © 2008 Eve Clark
All rights reserved.

ISBN: 1-4392-1011-X
ISBN-13: 9781439210116

Visit **www.booksurge.com** to order additional copies.

The Grocery Store Myth
The Good, The Bad, The Ugly

Eve Clark

ENDORSEMENTS

No matter how hard we try to do our best work and get along with others, we can't excel if we don't feel good. This starts with eating. "The Grocery Store Myth" is a fabulous book that shows how many foods in grocery stores, even vitamins, are not only weak in providing nutrition, they can actually make us sick. Thank you Eve for having the courage to reveal the truth and guide us to better health."

— Dr. Marcia Reynolds, PhD, author of *Outsmart Your Brain*

This book shows people how to look at their own eating habits and change to a healthier lifestyle. Thank you for providing a step by step explanation on how our food is raised, grown, prepared and sold in the grocery stores.

— Sue Dvoracek, RN

This book is a great eye-opener in getting across the real value of nutrition and how much you actually consume from the foods you're eating. It puts the emphasis on the *true* nutrition facts, what you're actually getting from the foods you eat, how to read labels, and what to make of them. Too often the consumer has the best intentions on making smart decisions, yet they are fooled by the tricky advertising that is allowed. The points brought up on how foods can truly harm you and what you can do about changing your diet and your grocery list, so you can live a better, healthier life is monumental. I encourage everyone to read this stimulating book!"

— Dr. Joe Brown, NMD

At one time or another, almost everyone has wanted to improve their eating habits and live a healthier lifestyle. The common grocery store can be confusing when it comes to food selection and achieving these goals. Clark provides a wonderful step by step guide which walks you around the grocery store, eliminating the confusion. She steers you towards healthy food choices in each department of the grocery store and explains why they are better choices. Clark also answers critical questions about how our food is prepared, supplied, and sold in grocery stores. This book is a must read!

— Dr. Melissa Dawahare, NMD, author of *House Call: How Ordinary People Have Extraordinary Health*

Our society has redefined the meaning of "food" for the past 40 years. It used to be simple. We bought food from the four basic food groups. Now, our food has additives and chemicals or has been modified in the growing process and we wonder why we are nutritionally imbalanced! Thanks to Eve Clark, we now have a kitchen manual to help us shop smarter so we can raise healthier families. Every shopper should have a copy of this book!

— Sherry Pitsch, Certified Herbalist

It's been a long time coming! Finally, a book to helps the average person sort out what's healthy, the difference in organic and what's good in our food. I wholeheartedly endorse this book as an educational and user-friendly guide for people who are increasing their awareness on the connection between our food and our health.

— Dr. Kareen O'Brien, NMD

Edited by
Roberta Proulx

Roberta Proulx is a Phoenix-based freelance writer and editor. She specializes in alternative health, fitness and family issues. In her spare time, she enjoys cooking and hiking with her husband and three boys.

Thank you Robbie for the excitement, enthusiasm and all the help you gave me with this book. You are a very special woman and a friend for life.

— Eve Clark

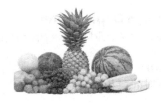

The Grocery Store Myth
The Good, The Bad, The Ugly

TABLE OF CONTENTS

Introduction: Birdseye View Of The Food We Eat — xi

Chapter 1 Fruits And Vegetables: Where Are They Grown — 1

Chapter 2 Deli Department: The Truth About Cold Cuts — 11

Chapter 3 Reading Labels, Dating, Canned Foods And Dents:
Tips On Reading The "Nutrition Facts" Value List On Products — 19

Chapter 4 Baked Goods:
The Key To Ingredients With Good Baking Tips — 37

Chapter 5 Meat, Poultry, Fish Department:
Hidden Secrets About How Our Food Is Raised — 51

Chapter 6 Cereal Aisle:
How Much Nutrition Do Cereals Have? — 73

Chapter 7 Snacks, Chips, And Crackers:
Where Do These Show Up On The Food Chart? — 81

Chapter 8 Frozen Foods:
Are These Healthier Than Fresh Foods? — 97

Chapter 9 Juice And Soft Drink Aisle:
How Bad Are These For Our Health? — 101

Chapter 10 Dairy And Egg Department:
Dairy And Eggs, Should We Avoid These Products? 117

Chapter 11 Conclusion:
Suggestions For A Healthier Life 125

References 137

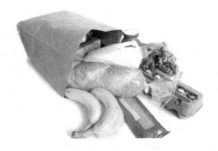

INTRODUCTION

GOOD FOOD, BAD FOOD, UGLY FOOD

The link between diet and health is nothing new. In 432 B.C., Hippocrates, the 'Father of Medicine,' is credited with saying, "Let thy food be thy medicine and thy medicine be thy food."

Fast forward to the 21st century, with mass-produced groceries that provide less nutrition and more entertainment for your taste buds than in the past. It is no wonder that more people suffer from chronic diseases than ever before. Your challenge is to find out whether the food and drink you consume is good for your health or not, then make the right choices for the health of you and your family. The time has come for medicine to return back to its roots: food.

Poor nutrition is not the only issue. Getting less than we need from food is one problem, getting unpleasant toxic bonuses in food is another. Modern groceries are laced with one dangerous additive after another. The double whammy of poor nutrition combined with toxic chemicals makes the advice of Dr. Elisa

Bandera, MD, PhD, most important when deciding what to eat, "...choose wisely."

The challenge now is that every grocery store offers thousands of food choices, with all kinds of ingredients that you must know about so you can choose the best ones for your health. Some become big news, like trans fats, to the extent that government regulators finally require information about them on food labels, and that cities and states are beginning to ban them from restaurants. However, the trans fat content in labels is highly misleading. Other ingredients, such as nitrites and aspartame, are economically so important to food manufacturers that they are kept under the public's radar, leaving a wake of toxic destruction that ruins the health of millions of people every year. There are many foods that add to good nutrition, and then there are the foods that rob you of your own wellbeing. Some toxins are more obvious, such as artificial flavors, colors, sweeteners, and preservatives. However, others are hidden or not so obvious.

The purpose of this book is to provide you with good knowledge about food choices so you can decide what is best for you and your family's health. Change lifelong habits if you must. Get your children back on the right track for good health, away from the sodas, candy, and packaged foods that seem to be everywhere, in schools and probably at home.

Eating and exercise habits begin when children are young. Early behaviors form foundations of health for the rest of their lives. Poor eating habits and physical inactivity during childhood set the stage for health problems as they grow up. Good eating habits and an active lifestyle are the key to longevity and good health. This is why conscientious shopping, with high nutrition and a low toxic load, can greatly reduce chronic diseases and create a healthy way of life.

Most Americans have changed their lifestyles to fast pace with fast food. Fifty years ago fresh fruits, vegetables, meats, eggs and dairy products arrived daily at grocery stores or markets. Stores stocked big barrels of fresh rice, beans and grains. They offered fresh baked breads without preservatives. Good choices were easier to make then. This definitely was a healthier way of life!

The purpose of this book is to help you determine which foods are good for you and which ones to avoid when you go to the grocery store. Some of the most important questions that are answered in this book include:

- What are the most toxic additives that you must avoid and what foods contain them? (Tricks of the food industry keep you in the dark.)
- Which fresh or packaged foods are most nutritious? (Fresh is not always the best.)
- Can any breakfast cereal be good for your health? (Understanding health claims on cereal boxes.)
- Exactly how bad are sodas? (Possibly the cause of more bad health than any other drink in human history.)
- What must you know before buying meat, fish, or poultry? (Big and juicy means hormones and antibiotics.)
- How can you interpret "Nutrition Facts" labels to be sure that you really get what you want? (Missing and misleading information makes this a big challenge.)
- Should you drink milk or not? (Bonus additives from bloated cows, plus the most nutrition-destroying process ever invented.)
- What is the latest on eggs – good or bad? (Eggs may be the best source of pure protein in the entire grocery store, if you make the right choices.)
- Can you snack your way to better health? (Chips and crackers are not your only options.)

Our lives have changed dramatically because of the food we eat. Basic nutrition has disappeared from our daily diets and has led to poor health. Toxic additives to make food look better, taste better, or last longer are more common than ever. One of the most worrisome health concern is overweight and obese adults and children. Shaping our lives with the right food can help reverse this huge problem.

More and more people would like to pursue healthier lifestyles and healthier eating habits. Today there is more awareness and emphasis on that foods that we consume and how they influence our overall health and wellness. If you look at people in other countries, they seem to be trimmer and more in shape than Americans. Many of these people have fewer health issues because they eat better, walk more, ride bikes and are overall more active.

What About the Food Pyramid?

The main theme of this book involves quality of food, the good, the bad, and the ugly. The importance of food groups for overall health, however, is the topic of a constant argument between those who recommend a low-fat diet vs. a low-carbohydrate diet. Fortunately, the best research on this controversy was completed recently, and the results favor fewer carbs with more of the right kind of fats for weight management and for lower cardiovascular risks. Compare these results with the pyramid of food groups provided by the U.S. Department of Agriculture:

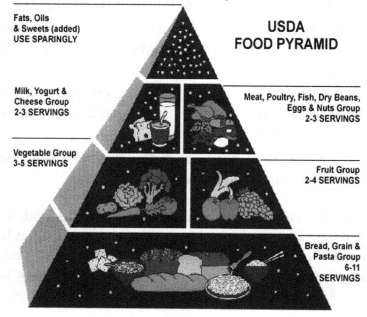

As you will learn later in this book, this is not as simple as it seems at first. Not all carbohydrates are created equal. The majority of the carbohydrate-rich foods at the bottom of this food pyramid, when consumed in the recommended proportions, will make you fat and ruin your health. On the other hand, your body requires a bigger dose of the right kinds of fats than you see at the top. In addition, guidelines for the consumption of dairy products are based on the political power of the dairy industry, not on any need for dairy products to be healthy. Regardless of what proportions that you select from each of these food groups, your health depends mostly on making sure that you choose high quality foods and avoid toxic and low quality foods as recommended in this book.

Grocery Store Guideline

When I began putting this book together, I wanted a unique guideline. So I used the format of a grocery store, corresponding to the aisles, to create each chapter.

- Chapter 1. Fruits and Vegetables. This chapter describes how fruits and vegetables are grown and harvested and how different methods influence the quality of food in the produce section. It also covers the use of pesticides and other chemicals that fruits and vegetables are exposed to before reaching the grocery store. You will learn some surprising information on how to choose products than can provide the best source of nutrition.

- Chapter 2. Deli Department. Yummy! Bacon with breakfast, ham sandwich for lunch, pepperoni pizza for dinner, hot dogs at the ballgame or picnic – all of these include examples of some of our favorite prepared foods, deli meats. Unfortunately, they offer almost no nutritional value and they contain one of the nastiest additives that you will ever find in food.

- Chapter 3. Understanding Package Labels. This chapter is dedicated to canned goods and food packaged in boxes.

Are the contents good if a can is damaged? What if the cans are outdated? Can preservatives in boxed food be bad for your health? This chapter is also about reading labels. How was the "Daily Value" on nutrition labels determined? This information can help you determine the real importance of contents in a package.

- Chapter 4. Baked Goods. What kind of flour is good for you and which ones should you steer away from? This chapter explains the differences in types of sugars and the substitutes used in our every day products.

- Chapter 5. Meat, Poultry, and Fish Department. This chapter describes how cattle, poultry, pork, chickens, and fish are raised and caught. I found stunning facts that will really surprise you about what happens to these foods before you buy them.

- Chapter 6. Cereal Aisle. Sweet and tasty. The biggest challenge in this aisle is to find healthy food among all of the empty calories in brightly colored boxes.

- Chapter 7. Chips and Crackers. The lowdown on chips, crackers, and other snack foods. Yes, you can make healthy choices on the bottom of the food pyramid.

- Chapter 8. Frozen foods. The secret about frozen foods nutritional value.

- Chapter 9. Juices and Soft Drink Aisle. The truth about soft drinks.

- Chapter 10. Dairy and Egg Department. A good way to start your mornings with a wholesome breakfast.

I own a nutrition store with my husband. One of the first questions I ask my customers is, "Did you take your vitamins today?" The majority of the answers are "Yes, and I took my 'One a Day' this morning." I wish this was a good answer but unfortunately it is not. Why is it not good enough and why should we take supplements with our food? In this book I explain why we pay more for groceries and get less nutrition from what we eat. You will read surprising facts about how our food is grown, raised and prepared.

Understanding food and nourishment is the first step in taking care of you. Determining the correct path for health and fitness can help you and your children live a longer and enjoyable life.

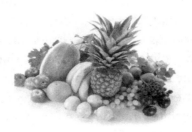

CHAPTER 1

FRUITS AND VEGETABLES

This chapter describes why fruits and vegetables are so important for healthy diets. It also details how they are grown and ultimately sold to our local grocery stores and how the handling of these products influences their nutritional value.

My mother always made sure I ate my fruits and vegetables. That was and still is a great recommendation for creating a healthy diet. Over the past 30 years or so, researchers have developed a solid base of science to back up what generations of mothers preached. We now know that eating plenty of fruits and vegetables can help you ward off heart disease and stroke, control blood pressure and cholesterol, avoid painful intestinal ailments like diverticulitis, and guard against cataracts and macular degeneration. In addition, fruits and vegetables are acclaimed as cancer-fighting foods. The latest research, though, suggests that the biggest payoff from eating fruits and vegetables is for the heart.

Signs posted in produce aisles, magazine ads, and schools recommend fresh food guidelines. These signs are supported in part by the National Cancer Institute. In fact, the initial five recommended servings a day of fruits and vegetables has changed. Some guidelines call for five to thirteen servings of fruits and vegetables a day, depending on one's caloric intake. For a person who needs 2,000 calories a day to maintain weight and health, this translates into nine servings, or four and one-half cups per day. U.S. nutrition officials are trying to help out. The U.S. Department of Agriculture (USDA) has created dietary guidelines to provide practical advice on how to give your child a healthy, balanced diet. The guidelines suggest that children eat more fruits, vegetables, and whole grains than what they are eating now. The recommendations are tailored for children based on age, gender, and exercise habits. You can find the guidelines that are appropriate for your child by logging on to the USDA's website on child nutrition programs at http://www.ers.usda.gov/Briefing/ChildNutrition.

Fruits and Vegetables vs. Cardiovascular Disease

The largest and longest study to date, done as part of the Harvard-based *Nurses' Health Study and Health Professionals Follow-up Study*, included almost 110,000 men and women whose health and dietary habits were followed for 14 years. Scientists found that the higher the average daily intake of fruits and vegetables, the lower the chances of developing cardiovascular disease. Those who averaged eight or more servings a day were 30% less likely to have had a heart attack or stroke.

Although all fruits and vegetables likely contribute to this benefit, green leafy vegetables are the most important overall. These include lettuce, spinach, Swiss chard and mustard greens, and cruciferous vegetables such as broccoli, cabbage, Brussels sprouts, bok choy, and kale.

High blood pressure is a primary risk factor for heart disease and stroke. Diet can be a very effective tool for lowering blood pressure. One of the most convincing associations between diet and blood pressure was found in the *Dietary Approaches to Stop Hypertension* (DASH) study. This study examined the effect on blood pressure of a diet that was rich in fruits and vegetables and low in fat. Researchers found that people with high blood pressure who followed this diet reduced their systolic blood pressure (the upper number of a blood pressure reading) by about 11 and their diastolic blood pressure (the lower number) by almost 6.

Eating more fruits and vegetables can also help lower cholesterol. In the National Heart, Lung, and Blood Institute's *Family Heart Study*, the 4,466 subjects consumed on average a little over three servings of fruits and vegetables a day. Men and women with the highest daily consumption (more than four servings a day) had significantly lower levels of LDL ("bad") cholesterol than those with lower daily consumption. How fruits and vegetables lower cholesterol is still something of a mystery. Soluble fiber in fruits and vegetables may block the absorption of cholesterol from food, or other mechanisms may be at work.

Fruits and Vegetables vs. Cancer

Fruits and vegetables may also protect against certain cancers. The International Agency for Research on Cancer, a part of the World Health Organization, recently completed a monumental review of the best research on fruits and vegetables vs. cancer. This 387-page work concludes that there is, "...evidence for a cancer-preventive effect of consumption of fruit and of vegetables for cancers of the mouth and pharynx, esophagus, stomach, colon-rectum, larynx, lung, ovary (vegetables only), bladder (fruit only), and kidney."

Keep in mind that this research looked at total fruit and vegetable consumption. However, specific fruits and vegetables may protect against specific types of cancer. For example, results from the *Health Professionals Follow-up Study* suggest that tomatoes may help protect men against prostate cancer. Lycopene, a pigment that gives tomatoes their red hue, could be involved in this protective effect. Furthermore, the increased consumption of tomato-based products (especially cooked tomato products) and other lycopene-containing foods may also reduce the occurrence or progression of prostate cancer.

Fruits and Vegetables vs. Gastrointestinal Disorders

One of the wonderful components of fruits and vegetables is their fiber. As fiber passes through the digestive system, it sops up water like a sponge and expands. This can calm the irritable bowel and, by triggering regular bowel movements, relieve or prevent constipation. The bulking and softening action of fiber also decreases pressure inside the intestinal tract and, in turn, may help prevent diverticulosis (the development of tiny, easily irritated pouches inside the colon) and diverticulitis (the often painful inflammation of these pouches).

Fruits, Vegetables, and Vision

Eating plenty of fruits and vegetables also keeps your eyes in good shape. You may have learned that carrots aid night vision. Other fruits and vegetables help prevent two common age-related eye diseases, cataract and macular degeneration. Cataract is the gradual clouding of the eye's lens. Macular degeneration is caused by cumulative damage to the macula, which is located in the center of the retina. This damage can be caused by free radicals generated by sunlight, cigarette smoke, air pollution and infections. Dark green leafy vegetables contain two pigments, lutein and zeaxanthin, which can snuff out free radicals before they harm the eye's sensitive tissues.

The Bottom Line: Recommendations for Fruit and Vegetable Intake

Fruits and vegetables are clearly an important part of a good diet. Almost everyone can benefit from eating more of them, but

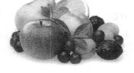

variety is as important as quantity. No single fruit or vegetable provides all of the nutrients you need to be healthy.

The key lies in eating a spectrum of different fruits and vegetables.

Some Basic Fruits And Vegetable Tips:
- Eat more fruits and vegetables. If you need 2,000 calories a day to maintain your weight and health, aim for at least nine servings (four and one-half cups) a day.
- Learn to appreciate many different fruits and vegetables. It's easy to get into a rut when it comes to the food you eat. Eat plenty of dark-green leafy vegetables, plus a variety of colored fresh produce. Include yellow, orange, and red. And don't forget cooked tomatoes and tomato-containing sauces.

Pesticides or No Pesticides

According to nutritionist Brenda Laizin, more pesticides are used in growing fruits and vegetable than ever before. Almost twenty different types of pesticides are available for use on food crops. Peaches seem to win the pesticide prize, but strawberries, nectarines, apples, bell peppers, celery, cherries, imported grapes, potatoes, spinach and raspberries are close behind. "Now it is important to keep in mind that even if you wash these fruits and vegetables, you will only reduce a little bit of the pesticides," says Lazin. This is because some pesticides are absorbed into the plant and others bind to the surface and are difficult to wash off.

So What's the Answer?

Laizin says, "You can adjust your eating habits by eating produce on the 'least contaminated' list." This list includes broccoli, cauliflower, asparagus, avocado, corn, kiwi, mangos, onions, bananas, papaya, pineapples and peas. You can also buy organic fruits and vegetables to avoid pesticides. Buying organic can, in some cases, cost twice as much as non-organic. However, if you shop in season, there's less difference in price.

Artificial vs. Natural Ripening

Years ago fruits were harvested only when ripe and then sent to market. Naturally ripened produce was fresh, tasty, and nutritious. Today it's a whole new ball game. Fruits are picked before they are ripe, stored in wholesale produce markets, and artificially ripened before being delivered to grocery stores.

Did you ever wonder where ripe oranges come from in July?

Artificial ripening is based on the use of a gas called ethylene, which is a naturally occurring plant hormone that causes ripening. As some fruits mature in nature, they produce this growth hormone to continue the ripening process. Without ethylene, fruits would not ripen. When fruits are harvested before they are ripe, then stored, they can be ripened artificially later by fumigation with ethylene gas. Examples of artificially ripened fruits include apples, avocados, bananas, citrus, dates, mangos, melons, papayas, pears, persimmons, pineapples, and tomatoes.

Ethylene Gas at the Grocery Store

A man made form of ethylene gas is used in ripening rooms to color fruits before they are moved to a regular cold storage room with other produce. Typical examples include bananas, tomatoes and avocados. Ethylene turns bananas yellow, tomatoes red and makes avocados soft and ready to eat.

Bananas, for example, are picked full-sized and green, before they are mature enough to produce their own ethylene for the natural ripening process. After their journey from Central or South America to North America, they are placed in special rooms, which are filled with ethylene to trigger the ripening process. The rooms are then aired out and the bananas sold, but they continue to ripen themselves by producing their own ethylene gas, going from the unripe green stage to the ready-to-eat yellow stage.

One problem with bananas is that they produce so much of their own ethylene that they become overripe quickly.

After picking, unripe citrus still has some green in the skin. Ethylene destroys the green chlorophyll pigment, allowing the underlying orange or yellow colors to show. This process is called <u>degreening.</u> The word degreening, simply means to get rid of the green color.

Green citrus (oranges, grapefruits, lemons) is not attractive to consumers. Consumers know that partially green citrus might not have full flavor. In order to convince consumers that navel oranges are tasty, for example, the color is changed from green to orange via the degreening process. Degreening rooms are used for this process. These rooms are totally insulated from the outside world and fully climate controlled for temperature, humidity, oxygen level, carbon dioxide level, and of course, ethylene gas level. Green navel oranges are stacked in the rooms and fumigated until they turn orange. The idea is that the fruit is made attractive to consumers by degreening. Unfortunately, the degreening process does nothing about the taste.

Ethylene gas is more than just a ripening agent for fruits. It also causes fruits to decay or over-ripen, it causes vegetables to decay and turn brown, and it causes flowers to bloom and wilt. Controlling ethylene gas after picking extends the shelf life of some fruits and vegetables, allowing them to be displayed at the grocery store for a much a longer period of time.

Ethylene is naturally produced by a number of vegetable crops. Potatoes, leafy and root vegetables produce varying amounts; cucumbers, okra, and peppers produce intermediate amounts. Honeydew melons and tomatoes are relatively high producers of ethylene.

When Ethylene Goes Too Far

Once a fruit or vegetable is delivered to stores, they continue to produce ethylene, which then becomes a problem. Decay and over-ripening ruins products. However, scientists have discovered chemicals that cancel out the effects of this gas. The most common one is called methylcyclopropene, which is sprayed onto fruits and vegetables to stop the ripening, browning, and decay. This allows fruits and vegetables to look good longer on the shelf.

Industrial Ethylene Gas and Food Crops

The commercial sources for this ethylene are natural gas and petroleum. An alternative source is used in some tomato greenhouses, where ethylene is made from alcohol. Man-made ethylene gas is a colorless gas with a sweet odor. Although it is flammable, the minimum flammable concentration is 3.1%, or about 200 times the concentration suggested for tomato ripening. This brings up a huge question. Which fruits and vegetables are you eating?

Symptoms of Ethylene Damage

You've seen the effects of ethylene gas damage many times:
- decay: (fresh produce and flower bulbs)
- russet spotting: (leafy vegetables and eggplants)
- yellowing: (cucumbers, broccoli and brussel sprouts)
- odor: (garlic and onions)
- wilting: (vegetables and cut flowers)
- scald and loss of crunch: (apples)
- rind breakdown: (citrus)

As markets expand across the country and around the world, preserving freshness in the presence of ethylene gas is one the biggest challenges in the fresh food industry. As a bonus benefit of research in this area, many ethylene control products also kill air-borne bacteria, viruses, sour rot, blue mold and brown rot fungi. The unanswered question about these chemicals is, what are they doing to your health?

Should Waxed Fruits and Vegetables Be Washed Before Eating?

Many fruits and vegetables are waxed before they are put on the produce shelf. The wax coating helps produce stay firm and crisp, and it also gives it an attractive shine. Wax won't hurt you, but the pesticides, herbicides, insecticides and sometimes the fungus sealed under wax can potentially harm you. So if your fruits aren't washed before eating, they could contain very small amounts of toxic chemicals. Washing produce can get rid of most of the harmful substances, according to a January 1998 study published in *Consumer Reports*. A little soap and a good brush will work to scrub off these chemicals.

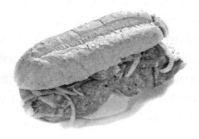

CHAPTER 2

DELI DEPARTMENT

Deli department include a wide variety of foods, from meats and cheeses to fruit and potato salads. This chapter, however, focuses on just one of these: cold cuts from meats and poultry.

Whole Piece Cuts

There are three types of cold cuts made from meat and poultry. The first type is cut from whole pieces such as roast beef, corned beef, or turkey breast. Whole cuts are exactly what they sound like, a section of meat or poultry that has been cooked, possibly flavored with salt, spices or sugars, and then sliced. Typically this is the more expensive type of cold cut.

Sectioned and Formed Meat Products

These are restructured meat products, such as multi-part turkey breasts or cooked hams. They are prepared from chunks or pieces of meat that are bonded together to form a single piece. The substances that bind these together are non-meat additives, meat emulsions and purified proteins. Typically they are produced by extracting the meat proteins (by adding salt and massaging or tumbling the meat, which brings these "sticky" proteins to the surface) or by adding non-meat proteins. Myosin is the major protein that is extracted. The meat becomes soft and pliable and is then shaped through molds or casings. Then it is cooked so the proteins will form a gel, thereby binding the chunks of meat together in a new shape.

Processed Meats (Sausages)

This is the majority of what we call 'cold cuts.' About 15% of all meat produced in the U.S. is used to make these meats; there are over 200 varieties. Sausage manufacturing includes any type of meat that is chopped, seasoned and formed into a symmetrical shape, such as bologna. There are two methods for preparing the ingredients: the emulsion method, where the meat is finely chopped so proteins can hold fat evenly throughout the mixture (examples are bologna, Vienna sausages, and hot dogs); and the non-emulsion method, which is typically used for coarser grinds. The same basic methods are used for sectioned and formed meat products, with no tumbling and massaging required. There are several meat sources for sausages, including beef, pork, mutton, veal, and poultry. Meat by-products are also used, including lips, tripe, pork stomachs and heart.

Curing Solutions

Curing solutions are injected into the meat with a needle or rubbed on the surface of raw meat. Curing solutions typically contain salt, sodium nitrate, and maybe sugar. Nitrate fuels action by bacteria that change it to nitrite, which causes light-colored substances in the meat to turn into a bright red pigment. This pigment is not very stable if the cured meat is exposed to light and oxygen in the display case. The pigment oxidizes and breaks down and turns the cured meat gray. Heat can also contribute to nitrite burns, which can induce the formation of a green pigment. The green/gray color of cured meats can also be triggered when the meat is contaminated by metals from molds or from smoke sticks. To stabilize the color, cured meats are often vacuum packaged. A common recommendation is to store the meat in the dark prior to display. Protecting cured meats from harmful visible and ultraviolet light, elevated temperatures and oxygen can help prevent cured meats from turning gray or green.

Sodium Nitrite

Sodium nitrite is used to prevent the growth of toxic bacteria called *Clostridium botulinum*, which can cause botulism in humans. It is used alone or in conjunction with sodium nitrate as a color fixative in cured meat and poultry products (bologna, hot dogs, and bacon). During the cooking process, nitrites combine with amines (naturally present in meat) to form cancer causing compounds. It is also suspected that nitrites can combine with amines in the human stomach to form similar compounds. These reaction products have been associated with cancer of the oral cavity, urinary bladder, esophagus, stomach and brain.

Deli Meats Are Highly Perishable

No food lasts forever, especially when it comes to cold cuts. While some of these products have natural or chemical preservatives to extend shelf life, packaged cold cuts only last three to five days once opened. Cold cuts sliced fresh from the deli last one to three days, if stored properly. Be sure to use an airtight plastic bag to store cold cuts and put them in the coldest part of the refrigerator.

Freshness dating of processed meats is a voluntary program and not mandated by the federal government. However, if there is a date on the package, by law, it must state clearly what the date signifies: "Sell by" date means nothing more than how long the store can display the product for sale. Never buy the product after this date.

"Best If Used By Date"

This date means that the flavor of the product will be at optimal taste and quality before the expired date. It has nothing to do with freshness or safety. Although luncheon meats comprise a segment of the larger processed- 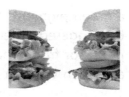 meats category, these products vary in composition, flavor and process. Pulverized meats, such as sausage, salamis, bologna and luncheon loaves, are either coarsely or finely chopped, cured, seasoned and, or smoked, heat-processed, or fermented and dried. The ingredients and process play a significant role in the texture and flavor of luncheon meats, and help characterize overall quality and shelf life.

Slicing Up Seasonings

Seasoned spices and other flavoring ingredients often characterize luncheon meats. "Bologna typically contains nutmeg, pimento, white pepper, mustard and sometimes coriander," says Jennifer Morgan, senior food technologist, Heller Seasonings & Ingredients Inc., Bedford Park, IL. "Salami uses a lot of garlic, cracked pepper, and possibly coriander, dried mustard and ginger. Liverwurst may contain mace, ginger, cardamom, bay and possibly marjoram. The flavor impact of whole, ground or cracked spices is a longer lasting flavor with an earthy impact. The finer the grind, the more immediate the impact," says Morgan. "Since spices may contain spoilage organisms, the best method of reduction of the organisms is irradiation, which does not harm the volatile oils in the spices, and therefore produces a better shelf life in the finished product." Spice extractives, oils and oleoresins are often used to give a higher and immediate flavor impact without visual effect, except oleoresin of paprika or capsicum, which provide the typical pink color in the finished product. In addition to spices, seasoning blends for luncheon meats also contain sweeteners and perhaps other flavoring ingredients. Typical sweeteners include sucrose, dextrose, corn syrup and or corn syrup solids. Some sweeteners provide benefits beyond simple sweetening capability. Sucrose and dextrose not only contribute to browning reaction for cooked products, but also play a role in the fermentation process for uncooked meats.

While luncheon meats are easy enough to consume, the development of such products is a bit more complex, requiring knowledge of federal regulations, food-safety issues, flavor-system development and meat-protein chemistry. No baloney here — just a bit of technical know-how to sink your teeth into.

Processed Meats Cause Cancer

Research in Sweden found that Swedes who ate three ounces of processed meat each day had a 15 percent greater chance of developing stomach cancer than those who consumed two ounces or less. Results of a seven year study by the Cancer Research Center of Hawaii and the University of Southern California reported in the Journal of the National Cancer Institute (2005;97:1458-65) that of 190,000 people, ages 45 to 75, those who ate the most processed meat (bacon, ham, and cold cuts) had a 68% higher risk of pancreatic cancer than those who ate the least. "Most" was defined as at least 0.6 ounce of processed meat, one ounce of beef or 0.3 ounce of pork per 1,000 calories consumed.

"The true cause of the heightened cancer risk is the widespread use of a carcinogenic precursor ingredient known as sodium nitrite by food processing companies," says Mike Adams, author of the just-published Grocery Warning manual. "Nearly all processed meats are made with sodium nitrite: breakfast sausage, hot dogs, jerkies, bacon, lunch meat, and even meats in canned soup products. Yet this ingredient is a precursor to highly carcinogenic nitrosamines (potent cancer-causing chemicals) that accelerate the formation and growth of cancer cells throughout the body. When consumers eat sodium nitrite in popular meat products, nitrosamines are formed in the body where they promote the growth of various cancers, including colorectal cancer and pancreatic cancer," says Adams. "Sodium nitrite is a dangerous, cancer-causing ingredient that has no place in the human food supply," he explains. The USDA actually tried to ban sodium nitrite in the 1970s, but was preempted by the meat processing industry, which relies on the ingredient as a color fixer to make foods look more visually appealing. "The meat industry uses sodium nitrite to sell more meat products at the expense of public health," says Adams. "And this new research clearly demonstrates the link between the consumption of processed meats and cancer." Pancreatic cancer isn't the only negative side effect of consuming processed meats such as hot dogs. Leukemia also skyrockets by 700% following the consumption of hot dogs. (Preston-Martin, S. et al. "N-nitroso compounds and childhood brain tumors: a case-control study." Cancer Res. 1982; 42:5240-5.) Other links between processed meats and disease are covered in detail in the Grocery Warning manual. Adams wrote Grocery Warning to warn consumers about the toxic, disease-causing ingredients found in everyday foods and groceries. "There are certain ingredients found in common grocery products that directly promote cancer, diabetes, heart disease, depression, Alzheimer's disease, osteoporosis and even behavioral disorders," Adams explains. His Grocery Warning manual covers them all, teaching readers how to prevent and even help reverse chronic diseases by avoiding the foods and food ingredients that cause disease. According to Adams, consumers can help reduce the cancer causing effects of sodium nitrite by consuming protective antioxidants before meals, such as vitamin C and vitamin E. But no vitamin offers 100% protection. The only safe strategy is to avoid sodium nitrite completely. Adams especially warns expectant mothers to avoid consuming sodium nitrite due to the greatly heightened risk of brain tumors in infants. Parents are also warned to avoid feeding their children products that contain sodium nitrite, including all popular hot dogs, bacon, jerkies, breakfast sausages and pizzas made with pepperoni or other processed meats. "Sodium nitrite is especially dangerous to fetuses, infants and children," says Adams. Sadly, nearly all school lunch programs currently serve school children meat products containing sodium nitrite. Hospital cafeterias also serve this cancer-causing ingredient to patients. Sodium nitrite is found in literally thousands of different menu items at fast food restaurants and dining establishments. "The use of this ingredient is widespread," says Adams, "and it is part of the reason we're seeing skyrocketing rates of cancer in every society that consumes large quantities of processed meats." Some companies are now offering nitrite-free and nitrate-free meat products, which are far healthier alternatives, but those products are difficult to find and are typically available only at health food stores or natural grocers. Consumers can look for "Nitrite-free" or "Nitrate-free" labels when shopping for meat products. They can also purchase fresh meats, which are almost never prepared with sodium nitrite. The new research on processed meats points to a chemical toxin as the cause of the increased cancer risk. "A heightened cancer risk of 67% is gigantic," warns Adams. This is clearly not due to macronutrient deficiencies. This is the kind of risk increase you only see with ingredient toxicity. Something in these processed meats is poisoning people, and the evidence points straight to sodium nitrite.

Nutrition Facts
Serving Size 1 cookie (28g)
Servings Per Container 15

Amount Per Serving	
Calories 120	Calories from Fat 45

	% Daily Value*
Total Fat 5g	8%
Saturated Fat 3g	15%
Cholesterol 25mg	8%
Sodium 100mg	4%
Total Carbohydrate 18g	6%
Dietary Fiber less than 1 gram	3%
Sugars 11g	
Protein 1g	

Vitamin A 4%	•	Vitamin C 0%
Calcium 2%	•	Iron 4%

*Percent Daily Values are based on a 2,000 calorie diet. Your daily values may be higher or lower depending on your calorie needs:

		Calories:	2,000	2,500
Total Fat		Less than	65g	80g
Saturated Fat		Less than	20g	25g
Cholesterol		Less than	300mg	300mg
Sodium		Less than	2,400mg	2,400mg
Total Carbohydrate			300g	375g
Dietary Fiber			25g	30g

Calories per gram:
Fat 9 • Carbohydrate 4 • Protein 4

CHAPTER 3

READING LABELS, DATING, CANNED FOOD AND DENTS

Have you found yourself in the supermarket with the best intention of making healthy selections, but didn't know where to start? The wrong shopping habits can severely hinder your health. The key to stocking your cupboards with healthy choices starts with understanding what you are filling them with. For many, decoding a package label can be as confusing as interpreting Latin. Knowing what to look for and what a label means will help you quickly decipher the difference between a good choice and what should be left on the shelf.

There are so many numbers, hard to read words, percentages, and facts that you almost feel dumbfounded trying to understand them. Confusion over nutrition can keep you from eating healthful quality foods. Reading food nutrition labels really doesn't have to be that intimidating. Once you take away the guesswork, reading food labels can be a quick and easy task that will require little time during your supermarket sweep.

Learning to read and understand food labels helps you compare nutritional values and enables you to buy more quality products that, in the long run, can even save you money! Three main parts of package labels provide information: 1) the front of the package, with name and basic contents plus one or more extra claims that are supposed to get your attention so you will buy it; 2) the ingredients list; 3) and, THE Nutrition Facts label on the side or back of the package

Front of the Package

Most package fronts are pretty straightforward. Some new claims have appeared on certain products over the years that take advantage of customer preferences rather than provide useful information. The non-cola sodas, for example, have always been caffeine free. The claim of "Caffeine Free" in big, bold lettering on the front of the bottle is a recent addition to the labels of these products. Lycopene, the red pigment in tomatoes, has become an important antioxidant in the eyes of consumers, so product labels on ketchup now point out that ketchup contains lycopene. Ketchup has always contained lycopene, so only the labels have changed. These are just two examples of labels that follow popular trends without really providing new benefits for the consumer. You can find lots of additional examples of this kind of useless product labeling throughout the grocery store.

Other claims are not so harmless. The biggest red flags are labels that claim to be sugar free, reduced sugar, zero trans fats, good for your heart, all natural, organic, all beef (or other meat), low fat, nonfat, low calorie, and whole wheat or grain. It is especially important for you to see through the hype of these kinds of claims by knowing what the real truth is behind them or how to understand the actual ingredients list on the side or back panel of the package. Government regulations for truth in labeling will not help you, since these regulations allow the food industry to slip in claims that allow manufacturers to get away with as much as possible. For example, the term "organic" can be applied to foods that have been sprayed with pesticides and herbicides or grown with chemical fertilizers. These chemicals just have to be applied below a certain allowable level. The term "all natural" for flavors and colors actually includes certain synthetic chemicals. In fact this is probably the most dangerous misleading claim on product labels throughout your grocery store, because it allows MSG (monosodium glutamate) to be hidden in hundreds of products without you knowing it. MSG is one of the most health-destroying additives ever included in packaged foods.

Think about this for a moment: What part of a cow can be put into a hot dog, lunch meat, or other processed meat and still be labeled as all beef? The answer is, any part. An all beef meat product could contain of fat, skin, intestine, cartilage, organ tissue, or anything else as long as it comes from somewhere on the cow. The only way to be sure what kind of meat you get is to get a whole cut from the animal.

Claims about being sugar free, reduced sugar, zero trans fats, good for your heart, low fat, nonfat, low calorie, and whole wheat or grain are common for many different kinds of products. You will read about examples of these later in the book, in chapters on baked goods, sodas, cereals, and dairy products. The following is a good general guide for what various terms on product labels mean, as defined in federal regulations.

- "Calorie free": Less than five calories per serving.
- "Low calorie": Forty calories or less per serving.

- "Reduced" or "less" calories: At least 25 percent fewer calories per serving when compared to a similar food.
- "Light" or "Lite": One-third fewer calories, or 50 percent less fat per serving.
- "Sugar free": Less than one-half gram of sugar per serving.
- "Reduced" or "less" sugar: At least 25 percent less sugar per serving, when compared with a similar food.
- "Fat free": Less than one-half gram of fat per serving.
- "Saturated Fat Free": Less than one-half gram of saturated fat per serving.
- "Low Saturated Fat": One gram or less per serving or not more than 15 percent of calories from saturated fat
- "Reduced" or "less" saturated fat: At least 25 percent less saturated fat per serving.
- "Sodium free": Less than five mg of sodium per serving.
- "Low sodium": One-hundred forty (140) mg or less per serving.
- "Very low sodium": Thirty-five (35) mg or less per serving.
- "Reduced" or "less" sodium: At least 25 percent less sodium per serving.
- "Low fat": Three grams or less per serving.
- "Reduced" or "less" fat: At least 25 percent less fat, when compared to a similar food.
- "Cholesterol free": Less than two mg of cholesterol per serving. "Low cholesterol": Twenty (20) mg or less of cholesterol per serving.
- "Reduced" or "less" cholesterol: At least 25 percent less cholesterol per serving.
- "Free," and other food terms. Less than one-half gram of fat per serving.

Here's the Low-Down on Using These Terms for Choosing Healthy Foods

Here's how you use these terms for choosing health foods. Healthy food must be low in fat, with limited cholesterol and sodium. Anything labeled "free" must only contain tiny amounts of the ingredient in each serving. For example, "trans fat free" or "fat free" products can have only 0.5 mg of trans fats or fat. "Cholesterol-free" foods can only have two milligrams of cholesterol and two grams of saturated fat. A serving of a food labeled "low sodium" can have a maximum of 140 milligrams of sodium. A serving of a "low cholesterol" food can have a maximum of 20 milligrams of cholesterol and two grams of saturated fat. One serving of a "low-fat" food can have a maximum of three grams of fat. A serving of a "low-calorie" food can have a maximum of 40 calories. A serving of a food labeled "reduced" must have 25% less of the ingredient (such as fat) than a serving of the regular version. One serving of a "light" food must have 50% less fat or one-third fewer calories than the regular version.

The most important and reliable information on the label can be found on the nutrition facts panel and the ingredient listing. The FDA sets specific rules for what food manufacturers can call light, low, reduced, one percent fat free.

Ingredients List

The fine print that includes all of the ingredients that have been added to a product are supposed to be included in the ingredients list. Furthermore, this list is supposed to be in order, starting with the most common ingredient and ending with the one with the least amount in the product. A simple example would be the following ingredients list for plain yogurt:

INGREDIENTS: CULTURED PASTEURIZED GRADE A NONFAT MILK, WHEY PROTEIN CONCENTRATE, PECTIN, CARRAGEENAN.

This product contains more cultured nonfat milk than anything else, because it is listed as the first ingredient. The ingredients of a true plain yogurt would stop there, but this product includes the additives that are listed after milk. For comparison, the following is a list ingredients for a similar product that contains added fruit:

> INGREDIENTS: CULTURED GRADE A REDUCED FAT MILK, APPLES, HIGH FRUCTOSE CORN SYRUP, CINNAMON, NUTMEG, NATURAL FLAVORS, AND PECTIN. CONTAINS ACTIVE YOGURT AND L. ACIDOPHILUS CULTURES.

Note that this product has been sweetened with high fructose corn syrup and flavored with cinnamon, nutmeg, and unexplained natural flavors. This product also has additional active culture, which is why it is listed here. This means that the original yogurt was boosted with additional yogurt culture.

The kinds of ingredients that appear in small print on the package of processed foods can give you an immediate idea about whether it might be good for you. In general, if the list is a long one, then you have to be especially careful in deciding whether your health would be better or worse for eating it. Take a look at this label and see what you think:

> 1 small bar 90 calories, 1.5g of fat, 95mg sodium, 1g fiber, 9g sugar, 1g protein)
> **INGREDIENTS:** Cereal (Rice, **Sugar**, Whole Grain Wheat, Wheat Gluten, Defatted Wheat Germ, Salt, **Wheat Flour**, **Malt Flavoring**, Maltodextrin, Riboflavin [Vitamin B2], Thiamin Hydrochloride [Vitamin B1]), **Corn Syrup**, Fruit Pieces, (**Sugar**, Blueberry, Juice Solids, Cranberries, Sunflower Oil), **Fructose, Sugar, Partially Hydrogenated Vegetable Oils** (Soybean and/or Cottonseed, and Palm Kernel), **Dextrose**, Nonfat Dry Milk, Natural and **Artificial Flavor**, **Sorbitol**, **Glycerin**, Soy Lecithin, Calcium Carbonate, Citric Acid, Salt, Niacinamide, **BHT (Preservative)**, Pyridoxine Hydrochloride (Vitamin B6).

It is difficult to quickly tell whether this is a good food or not. A detailed inspection of the ingredients shows sweeteners in seven places (sugars six times [sugar three times, dextrose, corn syrup, fructose], plus sorbitol). It also contains trans fats (partially hydrogenated oil from soybean, cottonseed, and/or palm kernel) and a synthetic preservative (BHT) among many other items.

Nutrition Facts

The Food and Drug Administration (FDA) requires all packaged food to contain accurate nutrition facts that pertain to serving size, calories per serving, fat, cholesterol, sodium, total carbohydrates, dietary fiber, sugars, protein and vitamins and minerals. The "Daily Value" of fat, cholesterol, sodium, total carbohydrates, dietary fiber, sugars and protein is also included on packaging labels. A good tip is to be aware of the percentage of total fats (including saturated fats), cholesterol, and sodium in each product. All of this information is supposed to be clearly presented in the "Nutrition Facts" label on every packaged product.

How important is it to read "Nutrition Facts" on food labels? Even though one glance at this label might send you into a slight panic, getting high quality products and real value for your money depends on you knowing the basic nutrition facts of your food. Here is a brief explanation of what each component of the Nutrition Facts label means in the following example for a box of macaroni and cheese.

The information in the main or top section can vary with each food product; it contains product-specific information (serving size, calories, and nutrient information). The bottom part contains a footnote with Daily Values (DVs) for 2,000 and 2,500 calorie diets. This footnote provides recommended dietary information for important nutrients, including fats, sodium and fiber. The footnote is found only on larger packages and does not change from product to product.

> Serving Size 1 cup (228g)
> Servings Per Container 2

The first place to start when you look at the Nutrition Facts label is the serving size and the number of servings in the package. Serving sizes are standardized to make it easier to compare similar foods; they are provided in familiar units, such as cups or pieces, followed by the metric amount, e.g., the number of grams.

> **Amount Per Serving**
> **Calories** 250   Calories from Fat 110

Calories provide a measure of how much energy you get from a serving of this food. Many Americans consume more calories than they need without meeting recommended intakes for a number of nutrients. The calorie section of the label can help you manage your weight (i.e., gain, lose, or maintain). Remember: the number of servings you consume determines the number of calories you actually eat (your portion amount). In the example, there are 250 calories in one serving of this macaroni and cheese. How many calories from fat are there in ONE serving? Answer: 110 calories, which means almost half the calories in a single serving come from fat. What if you ate the whole package content? Then, you would consume two servings, or 500 calories, and 220 would come from fat. The federal General Guide to Calories provides a general reference for calories when you look at a Nutrition Facts label.

This guide is based on a 2,000 calorie diet, as follows: 40 Calories is low, 100 Calories is moderate, 400 Calories or more is high.

Total Fat 12g	18%
Saturated Fat 3g	15%
Trans Fat 3g	
Cholesterol 30mg	10%
Sodium 470mg	20%

Look at the top of the nutrient section in the sample label. It shows you some key nutrients that impact on your health and separates them into two main groups. The nutrients listed above are the ones Americans generally eat in adequate amounts, or even too much. Eating too much fat, saturated fat, *trans* fat, cholesterol, or sodium may increase your risk of certain chronic diseases, like heart disease, some cancers, or high blood pressure.

Dietary Fiber 0g	0%
Vitamin A	4%
Vitamin C	2%
Calcium	20%
Iron	4%

Most Americans don't get enough dietary fiber, vitamin A, vitamin C, calcium, and iron in their diets. Eating enough of these nutrients on the label above can improve your health and help reduce the risk of some diseases and conditions. For example, getting enough calcium may reduce the risk of osteoporosis, a condition that results in brittle bones as you get older. Eating a diet high in dietary fiber promotes healthy bowel function. Additionally, a diet rich in fruits, vegetables, and grain products that contain dietary fiber, particularly soluble fiber, and low in saturated fat and cholesterol may reduce the risk of heart disease.

Note the * used after the heading "%Daily Value" on the Nutrition Facts label. It refers to the Footnote in the lower part of the nutrition label, which tells you "%DVs are based on a 2,000 calorie diet." This statement must be on all food labels. But the remaining information in the full footnote may not be on the package if the size of the label is too small. When the full footnote does appear, it will always be the same. It doesn't change from product to product, because it shows recommended dietary advice for all Americans—it is not about a specific food product.

Look at the amounts circled in the footnote—these are the Daily Values (DV) for each nutrient listed and are based on public health experts' advice. DVs are recommended levels of intakes. DVs in the footnote are based on a 2,000 or 2,500 calorie diet. Note how the DVs for some nutrients change, while others (for cholesterol and sodium) remain the same for both calorie amounts.

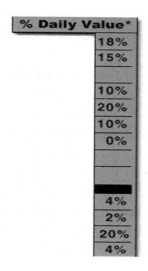

The % Daily Values (%DVs) are based on the Daily Value recommendations for key nutrients but only for a 2,000 calorie daily diet—not 2,500 calories. You, like most people, may not know how many calories you consume in a day. But you can still use the %DV as a frame of reference whether or not you consume more or less than 2,000 calories. The %DV helps you determine if a serving of food is high or low in a nutrient. Note: a few nutrients, like trans fat, do not have a %DV—they will be discussed later. Do you need to know how to calculate percentages to use the %DV? No, the label (the %DV) does the math for you. It helps you interpret the numbers (grams and milligrams) by putting them all on the same scale for the day (0-100%DV). The %DV column doesn't add up vertically to 100%. Instead each nutrient is based on 100% of the daily requirements for that nutrient (for a 2,000 calorie diet). This way you can tell high from low and know which nutrients contribute a lot, or a little, to your <u>daily</u> recommended allowance (<u>upper or lower</u>).

Now look at the example below for another way to see how the Daily Values (DVs) relate to the %DVs and dietary guidance. For each nutrient listed there is a DV, a %DV, and dietary advice or a goal. If you follow this dietary advice, you will stay within public health experts' recommended upper or lower limits for the nutrients listed, based on a 2,000 calorie daily diet.

Examples of DVs versus %DVs
Based on a 2,000 Calorie Diet

Nutrient	**DV**	**%DV**	**Goal**
• Total Fat	65g	= 100%DV	Less than
• Sat Fat	20g	= 100%DV	Less than
• Cholesterol	300mg	= 100%DV	Less than
• Sodium	2400mg	= 100%DV	Less than
• Total Carbohydrate	300g	= 100%DV	At least
• Dietary Fiber	25g	= 100%DV	At least

Upper Limit - Eat "Less than" the nutrients that have "upper daily limits" are listed first on the footnote of larger labels and on the example above. Upper limits means it is recommended that you stay below - eat "less than" – the Daily Value nutrient amounts listed per day. For example, the DV for Saturated fat is 20 g. This amount is 100% DV for this nutrient. What is the goal or dietary advice? Eat "less than" 20 g or 100%DV for the day.

Lower Limit - Eat "At least" Now look at the section where dietary fiber is listed. The DV for dietary fiber is 25g, which is 100% DV. This means it is recommended that you eat "at least" this amount of dietary fiber per day. The DV for Total Carbohydrate (section in white) is 300g or 100%DV. This amount is recommended for a balanced daily diet that is based on 2,000 calories, but can vary, depending on your daily intake of fat and protein.

Dented Cans

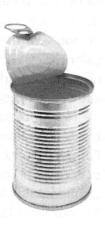

Products in slightly dented cans can be consumed as long as there are no leaks and the product appears wholesome. Do not consume products from severely dented, leaking, or swollen cans or jars. Avoid canned foods that are swollen or bulging, leaking, rusted or dented at the seam or rim. Denting at the seam or rim may allow air into the can, potentially exposing the contents to bacteria and other pathogens. This can cause a food and health safety risk. When air enters a can, bacteria can start growing, and this can be very dangerous. Do not use cans with sharp dents. Stores should throw away cans dented in dangerous ways. For more information refer to http://www.foodsafetynetwork.com.

Are Smashed Boxes of Cereal Safe?

Before it is made available for sale, each box of cereal is inspected to ensure that the plastic bag inside of the cardboard box is airtight and not punctured. The outside cardboard box will sometimes need to be torn in order to check the safety of the cereal, so on occasion you will find a taped box. The cereal inside of the airtight bag is perfectly safe to eat.

Expiration Dates

What about the labels on the food items sold at discount grocers? According to the Food Safety and Inspection Service of the U.S Department of Agriculture, product dating is not required by federal regulation. The exception is infant formula and some baby foods. The labels that you find on different products are there to help the consumer, but I have found that more often than not expiration dates are misleading.

Food Product Dating

There is no uniform or universally accepted system used for food dating in the United States. Although dating of some foods is required by more than 20 states, there are areas of the country where much of the food supply has some type of open date and other areas where almost no food is dated.

What is Dating?

Open Dating on a food product is a date stamped on a product's package to help the store determine how long to display the product for sale. It can also help the purchaser to know the time limit to purchase or use the product at its best quality. Open dating is not a safety date. After the date passes, the product should still be safe for a short time, if handled properly. If a product has a "use-by" date, follow that date. If a product has a "sell-by" date or no date, cook or freeze the product by the "sell-by date, or check with the manufacturer before consuming the product.

What Types of Food are Dated?

Open dating is found primarily on perishable foods such as meat, poultry, eggs and dairy products. "Closed" or "coded" dating might appear on shelf-stable products such as cans and boxes of food.

Types of Dates

- "Sell-By" date tells the store how long to display the product for sale. You should buy the product before the date expires.
- "Best if Used By (or Before)" date is recommended for best flavor or quality. It is not a purchase or safety date.
- "Use-By" date is the last date recommended for the use of the product while at peak quality. The date has been determined by the manufacturer of the product.
- "Closed or coded dates" are packing numbers for use by the manufacturer.

Foods Can Develop Odors

When food ages or appearance change due to bacteria it should not be used for quality reasons. If foods are mishandled, food-borne bacteria can grow and cause food-borne illness before or after the date on the package. For example, if hot dogs are taken to a picnic and left out for several hours, they wouldn't be safe if used afterwards even if the date hasn't expired. Other examples of potential mishandling are products that have been defrosted at room temperature more than two hours, cross contaminated, or handled by people who don't use proper sanitary practices. Make sure to follow the handling and preparation instructions on the label to ensure top quality and safety.

Dating Formula and Baby Food

Federal regulations require a "use-by" date on product labels of infant formula and baby food under FDA inspection. The formula or food must contain not less than the quantity of each nutrient as described on the label. Formula must maintain an acceptable quality to pass through an ordinary bottle nipple. If stored too long, formula can separate and clog the nipple.

What Do Can Codes Mean?

A can must exhibit a packing code to enable tracking of the product in interstate commerce. This enables manufacturers to rotate their stock as well as to locate their products in the event of a recall. These codes, which appear as a series of letters and/or numbers, might refer to the date or time of manufacture. They aren't meant for the consumer to interpret as "use-by" dates. There is no book which tells how to translate the codes into dates.

Open Calendar Date

A Can may also display "open" or calendar dates. Usually these are "best if used by" dates for peak quality. In general, high-acid canned foods such as tomatoes, grapefruit and pineapple can be stored on the shelf 12 to 18 months. Low-acid canned foods such as meat, poultry, fish and most vegetables will keep 2 to 5 years if the can remains in good condition and has been stored in a cool, clean, dry place.

Dates on Egg Cartons

Use of either a "sell-by" or "Expiration" (EXP) date is not federally required, but may be state required, as defined by the egg laws in the state where the eggs are marketed. Some state egg laws do not allow the use of a "sell-by" date. Many eggs reach stores only a few days after the hen lays them. Egg cartons with the USDA grade shield on them must display the "pack date" (the day that the eggs were washed, graded, and placed in the carton). The number is a three-digit code that represents the consecutive day of the year starting with January 1 as 001 and ending with December 31. When a "sell-by" date appears on a carton bearing the USDA grade shield, the code date may not exceed 45 days from the date of pack. Always purchase eggs before the "sell-by" or "EXP" date on the carton. After you bring the eggs home, refrigerate them in the coldest part of the refrigerator, not in the door. For best quality, use eggs within 3 to 5 weeks of the date you purchase them. If the "sell-by" date expires during that length of time, the eggs are still perfectly safe to use.

UPC or Bar Codes

Universal Product Codes appear on packages as black lines of varying widths above a series of numbers. They are not required by regulation but manufacturers print them on most product labels because scanners at supermarkets can "read" them quickly to record the price at checkout. Bar codes are used by stores and manufacturers for inventory purposes and marketing information. When read by a computer, they can reveal information such as the manufacturer's name, product name, size of product and price. The numbers are not used to identify recalled products.

Storage Times

Since product dates aren't a guide for safe use of a product, how long can the consumer store the food and still use it at top quality? Follow these tips:

- Purchase the product before the date expires.
- If perishable, take the food home immediately after purchase and refrigerate it promptly. Freeze it if you can't use it within times recommended on chart.
- Once a perishable product is frozen, it doesn't matter if the date expires because foods kept frozen continuously are safe indefinitely.
- Follow handling recommendations on product.

Why are there No Ingredient Statements on Some Products, Such as Coffee?

Some products only have one ingredient and therefore would not carry an ingredient statement. You can use the percent daily values number to determine whether a food is high or low in a nutrient. A food is low in a nutrient if it provides less than five percent of the nutrient. A food is high in a nutrient if it provides more than twenty percent of the nutrient.

Why Are Some Ingredients Not Listed At All?

Caffeine is a good example of an ingredient in coffee, colas, and certain teas. However, most of these products say nothing on the label about caffeine because it occurs naturally in these plants. Since anything from a plant or animal can contain thousands of natural products, none of them have to be listed on the ingredients list. Only specific ingredients that have been added later must be listed. This means that, when you find sugar or caffeine in an ingredient list, it was added in later. Colas with caffeine on the label not only contain caffeine from the cola nut, they contain extra caffeine that was added to the final product formula.

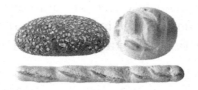

CHAPTER 4
BAKED GOODS

Baking and cooking goods are most commonly thought of as white foods because they contain so much flour and sugar. How can you determine which of these kinds of foods are best for your health? The answers come partly from knowing the differences between simple and complex carbohydrates, flours and sugars, and natural vs. artificial sweeteners.

Types of Flour

Many people think of flour in terms of wheat flour, although all-purpose "bleached" flour is used most frequently. In fact, flour can be ground from a variety of nuts and seeds. Some types of flours available are: amaranth, arrowroot, barley, buckwheat, chickpea, corn, kamut, nuts, oats, potato, quinoa, rice, rye, soy, spelt, tapioca, teff, wheat, and vegetables.

Types of typical flours:

- Unbleached flour is simply not as white as bleached.
- Whole-wheat flour is brown in color, and is derived from the complete wheat kernel (the bran and germ). When whole wheat flour is used in bread baking, it gives a nutty flavor and a denser texture compared to all-purpose flour.
- Bread flour is higher in protein than bleached flour.
- Cake flour has the least amount of gluten. Cake flour often comes bleached, which gives it a bright, white appearance.
- Pastry flour has low gluten content, although it contains a bit more than cake flour. Pastry flour is made from soft wheat flour.
- High-gluten flour is milled from hard wheat and has high protein content. Spelt flour contains gluten. It can, however, be tolerated by some people with gluten allergies. When making bread with spelt flour, the bread is not kneaded as long as other breads, since the gluten is not as durable as that of other wheat flowers. Spelt flour may be frozen if not used right away.

Enriched Flour

According to the FDA, a pound of flour must have the following quantities of nutrients to qualify as enriched flour:

- 2.9 milligrams of thiamin
- 1.8 milligrams of riboflavin
- 24 milligrams of niacin
- 0.7 milligrams of folic acid
- 20 milligrams of iron

The first four nutrients are B vitamins. Calcium may also be added at a minimum of 960 milligrams per pound. Enriching is necessary because the processing used to make white flour destroys some nutrients originally present in the whole grain. The reason that enriched flour is called "enriched" as opposed to "fortified" is because nutrients are added for the purpose of replacing those lost during flour processing, as opposed to introducing nutrients that were never in the food originally.

Carbohydrates

Carbohydrates appear in many forms in many foods. Carbohydrates belong to a group of nutrients containing carbon atoms that have been hydrated by adding water molecules. Carbohydrates are actually built of sugar molecules, called saccharides.

Carbohydrates include sugars, starches, and fiber. Both sugars and starches are broken down by the body into a simple sugar, glucose. Glucose molecules circulate in the bloodstream, supplying cells with fuel on an as-needed basis. Extra glucose is converted into glycogen, which is stored in muscles and the liver. If the body is already storing enough glycogen, glucose gets changed into fat. Your body prefers to burn glucose or glycogen for energy, but when these reserves are depleted it draws on fat, the reserve fuel.

Carbohydrates are an important part of the diet, since they provide calories that your body uses for energy to grow, to work, and to repair itself. Simple carbohydrates are those that contain only one or two saccharides. One example of a simple sugar is fructose, which is called fruit sugar because it is so common in fruits. It is the sweetest of all the sugars. If the carbohydrate contains two sugar units, it is known as a disaccharide. Common table sugar, sucrose, is a disaccharide.

Complex carbohydrates are known as polysaccharides. As a general rule, complex carbohydrates such as starches are associated with more nutrition, since they are usually part of foods that contain a variety of other nutrients and not a lot of fat.

Starches, like simple sugars, are broken down into glucose by the body. Starches take longer to digest than simple sugars, so they don't cause blood sugar fluctuations the way simple sugars do.

Fiber is also a complex carbohydrate. However, human intestines do not contain the enzymes necessary to break down the fiber's long carbohydrate necklace into individual sugar molecules so that it can be absorbed in the bloodstream. Carbohydrates don't count as calories in the diet unless they are burned for energy, so fiber is really a calorie-free food. Fiber in a food slows the digestion of other carbohydrates, especially soluble fibers from citrus fruits, oats, and legumes. The extra fiber in whole grains also slows the digestion and absorption of sugar, which explains why whole grains in cereal are digested more slowly than high-carb pasta.

Satisfying Carbs

Beginning a meal with a complex carbohydrate food, such as pasta, and eating it slowly will lessen your craving for fats during the rest of the meal. You'll start to feel full and won't want as much of the higher-fat foods. So use pasta (with low-fat sauce) to curb overeating. Complex carbohydrates are found in grains, vegetables, and legumes that provide vitamins, minerals, and fiber as well as energy. You get a lot of nutritional bang for your buck with complex carbs.

Rating Sugars

There are many different kinds of sugar besides the familiar white grains in the sugar bowl. Nutritionally speaking, there is no such thing as a bad sugar, since all digestible sugars provide energy to the body. It doesn't matter to an individual cell whether the glucose it is using for fuel entered the body as a starch or as a sugar. Yet, simple and complex carbohydrates behave differently in the body and are part of different nutritional packages. The best carbs are those that provide both a steady supply of energy as well as a other nutrients the body needs. The worst carbs come in packages with few other nutrients and cause blood sugar to be unstable.

Next Best Sugars

Fructose is a single saccharide rather than a complex carbohydrate. It comes from fruit that also contains important nutrients and fiber. Fruits provide quick energy, but do not excite the blood sugar roller coaster because they also contain fiber that slows absorption of the simple sugars. Unlike the simple sugar glucose that quickly enters the bloodstream, fructose has to go to the liver before it is released into the bloodstream and carried to the body's cells.

Caution Sugars

Why do some sugars merit the label "junk sugars?" After refined sugars rush into the bloodstream, blood sugar levels rise, pressuring the pancreas to release insulin, the hormone needed to escort these sugars into the body's cells. Lots of insulin helps the sugar get used up rapidly, but then blood sugar levels plunge. The body hits a sugar low, also known as hypoglycemia or "sugar blues." Now, just as insulin was released when the blood sugar was too high, other hormones are released when the blood sugar is too low. These stress hormones are supposed to restore the blood sugar to normal levels, so they squeeze stored sugar from the liver, sending the blood sugar back up. These adjustments work better in some people than in others and better in some circumstances than in others. Sugar-sensitive individuals experience the ups and downs of blood sugar levels as a roller-coaster ride, and their moods and behavior go up and down with their blood sugar.

Maltose is composed of two molecules of glucose and is the sugar found in barley malt and some cereals. Maltose in beer causes a rapid rise in blood sugar. Corn syrup is a sugar extracted from corn. Being extracted from corn doesn't make it any healthier than ordinary table sugar. Syrups are really sugar concentrates and one tablespoon of syrup, corn or maple, contains about twice the amount of calories as a tablespoon of granulated sugar. While syrups do contain traces of a few minerals, such as calcium, phosphorus, iron, potassium, and sodium, they essentially have the same nutritional value as sugar. Because corn syrup is cheap to produce, it is the most popular sweetener for beverages, and even some juices. Corn syrup has high calorie content and it is seldom found in diet drinks. High-fructose corn syrup contains 40 to 90 percent fructose. It is a popular and inexpensive sweetener in cereals and sodas. Molasses is thick syrup, a byproduct of the sugar-refining process. Yet, unlike ordinary table sugar, molasses contains other valuable nutrients besides carbohydrates. The darker the molasses, the greater its nutritional value. Blackstrap molasses, for example, is a valuable source of calcium, iron and potassium, and also contains traces of B-vitamins. Brown sugar is simply ordinary table sugar made brown by adding molasses. Brown sugar contains a trace more nutritional value than white sugar, but not enough to make it any more valuable as a source of nutrients. "Raw" sugar is more a marketing gimmick than a real nutritional food. The term "raw" implies a more natural sugar. Yet, raw sugar is nothing more than crystallized, refined white sugar with a touch of molasses left in.

Harmful Sugars

Certain sugars belong in the same category as the fake fats. They contribute no essential nutrients to the body, and they actually may harm.

Junk sugars in soft drinks also deplete the body of nutrients. High doses of sugar and artificial sweeteners remove calcium, leading to weaker bones, or osteoporosis. Junk sugars can deposit calcium in the kidneys leading to kidney stones. The phosphoric acid present in many soft drinks further robs the body of calcium by increasing loss of magnesium and calcium.

These high doses of sugar also fill children up, so they tend to eat less of the nutritious foods. They drink cola with a meal instead of milk, or they reach for other junk food to go with the empty calories in their soda. They choose high-fat fast-food since television has made the junk cola along with a junk sandwich the American nutritional norm.

Natural Sweeteners That Can Bloat You

Some fruits contain sweet sugar-like substances called sugar alcohols. One of these is sorbitol, which can cause gas, bloating, and diarrhea. Plums are the fruits with the highest amount of sorbitol. This is why prunes, which are dried plums, act like a laxative. The next highest sorbitol containing fruits are pears and cherries. Peaches and apples contain a tiny bit of sorbitol, and citrus fruits contain none at all. Sugar-free gums, candies, and other low-calorie food are often sweetened with sorbitol, which is why eating them in excess can cause a reaction in your body much like eating prunes.

Packaged Bakery Goods and Sugar

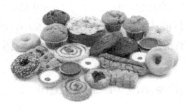

The combination of white sugar, white flour, and hydrogenated shortening makes bakery goods empty packages of nutrition. Most sweet snacks, such as cupcakes and doughnuts, contain all three of these factory-made foods. Instead, look for baked goods made with whole grains that contain no hydrogenated oils, and are sweetened with fruit concentrates.

How Sugar Harms

The complex carbohydrates found in vegetables, grains, and fruits are good for you; the simple sugars found in sodas, candies, icings, and packaged treats can do harm, at least when eaten in excess. It is as simple as that. Excess sugar depresses immunity. Studies have shown that downing 75 to 100 grams of a sugar solution (about 20 teaspoons of sugar, or the amount contained in two average 12-ounce sodas) can suppress the body's immune responses.

Simple sugars, including glucose, table sugar, fructose, and honey caused a fifty percent drop in the ability of white blood cells to engulf bacteria. In contrast, ingesting a complex carbohydrate solution (starch) did not lessen the ability of white blood cells to engulf bacteria. Immune suppression was most noticeable two hours post-ingestion, but the effect was still evident five hours after ingestion. This research has practical implications, especially for teens and college students who tend to overdose on sodas containing caffeine and sugar while studying for exams or during periods of stress. Stress suppresses immunity, so these sugar-users are setting themselves up to get sick at a time when they need to be well.

An Overdose of Sugar

Eating or drinking 100 grams (eight tablespoons) of sugar, the equivalent of two and one half twelve ounce cans of soda, can reduce the ability of white blood cells to kill germs by 40 percent. The immune-suppressing effect of sugar starts less than thirty minutes after ingestion and may last for five hours.

Alternative Sweeteners

Cinnamon is a sweet spice, and a small amount goes a long way. Two teaspoons of cinnamon can change a tart apple pie to a sweet one, lessening the amount of sugar needed. As an added nutritional perk, a teaspoon of cinnamon contains 28 milligrams of calcium and traces of B-vitamins, fiber, and iron. Try these herbs and spices to accent the flavor in foods: mint, cloves, anise, and ginger. A twist of lemon gives flavor to most beverages, including plain water. Use fruit toppings such as crushed pineapple, applesauce, strawberries, or blueberries instead of syrup on pancakes and waffles. Sprinkle cinnamon or nutmeg on fruit to bring out the fruit's natural sweetness. Plain yogurt flavored with fresh fruit is less sweet and contains healthier sugars than syrupy fruit preserves. Frozen fruits packed in water or natural juices are much better than those packed in syrups. You may have to experiment to discover how low you can go with sugar and still have a flavor that you find acceptable. Instead of sugar, substitute honey or molasses.

Artificial Sweeteners

Aspartame, like saccharin, was originally developed as a sugar substitute for diabetics, but the manufacturer soon discovered a huge market in a calorie-conscious society.

Artificial sweeteners do not typically satisfy a body that is craving sweets or carbohydrates. In fact, they may condition the taste buds to accept sweet flavors to the point that sweetener-users want more sweeteners rather than less. The more sweets you eat, the more your taste buds get used to the sweet taste and the more sweetener you require to satisfy your cravings.

Some scientists are concerned about biochemical quirks of artificial sweeteners. The sweetener aspartame ("Nutrasweet") is basically a combination of two common amino acids: aspartic acid and phenylalanine. One of the drawbacks of using this sweetener is that it is unstable when it gets warm. That is why you are not supposed to cook or bake with it. When aspartame warms to body temperature, one of the byproducts of its breakdown is methanol. Methanol is a poison that is metabolized by the liver into formaldehyde (a deadly neurotoxin, carcinogen, mutagen, and teratogen – meaning that it can cause birth defects). Methanol is also a cumulative liver toxin whose symptoms include headaches, tinnitus, shooting pains, memory lapses, numbness and nerve inflammation. Heavy use of aspartame can even cause symptoms of multiple sclerosis. Further prominent symptoms are blurred vision, retinal damage and blindness. Another problem with artificially-sweetened drinks is that people tend to drink a lot of them. The calories in a sugar-containing soda can satisfy the appetite. When you drink an artificially-sweetened beverage, your body may want more, further confusing your brain to want more.

Sucralose

Sucralose, also known by its trade name, Splenda, is 600 times sweeter than sugar. Sucralose tastes like sugar because it is made from table sugar. But it cannot be digested, so it adds no calories to food. Because sucralose is so much sweeter than sugar, it is bulked up with maltodextrin, a starchy powder, so it will measure more like sugar. It has good shelf life and doesn't degrade when exposed to heat. Numerous studies have shown that sucralose does not affect blood glucose levels, making it an option for diabetics.

After reviewing more than 110 animal and human safety studies conducted over 20 years, the FDA approved it in 1998 as a tabletop sweetener and for use in products such as baked goods, nonalcoholic beverages, chewing gum, frozen dairy desserts, fruit juices, and gelatins. The FDA has amended its regulation to allow sucralose as a general-purpose sweetener for all foods.

Sugar Alcohols

Though not technically considered artificial sweeteners, sugar alcohols are slightly lower in calories than sugar and do not promote tooth decay or cause a sudden increase in blood glucose. They include sorbitol, xylitol, lactitol, mannitol, and maltitol and are used mainly to sweeten sugar-free candies, cookies, and chewing gums. The FDA classifies some of these sweeteners as "generally recognized as safe" and others as approved food additives.

Other Natural Sweeteners

There are other natural sweeteners available, but these are variations of table sugar and contain about the same amount of calories. These products include honey, molasses, evaporated cane juice, rice syrup, barley malt, and fructose. Regardless of the sweetener you use, you can help your taste buds regain their sensitivity to sweetness by simply eating foods that are less sweet.

Stevia

The sweet tasting stevia leaf is derived from a South American shrub. In 2008, Jim May challenged an FDA decision and won the right to distribute stevia as a sweetener. His product, called SweetLeaf Sweetener, unlike most food supplements, contains no calories or carbohydrates and does not raise blood sugar levels, making it safer, for example, for diabetes patients.

Stevia is 200–300 times sweeter than table sugar. "My experience is that the herbal powder is very safe and is one of only a few substitutes that help control sugar spikes in the blood," says May. According to some research, it may actually lower blood sugar levels. However, this research has yet to be confirmed and contradictory results make any conclusions premature. Stevia and its extracts are extremely heat stable in a variety of everyday cooking and baking situations.

The Sweetness of Honey

Honey has been renowned as a source of energy and nutrition since humans discovered bees. The Romans regarded honey as "nectar of the gods," and Greek athletes energized themselves with honey before entering the arena. Egyptians put honey in tombs as food for the afterlife. In fact, honey was used as a sweetener for centuries before humans learned how to extract sugar from sugarcane or beets. The biblical Promised Land "flowed with milk and honey," and Hippocrates in his writings on the care and cure of the patient extolled the nutritional virtues of honey. In short, history regards honey as man's original and most natural sweetener.

Trans Fats

Trans fats (also known as trans fatty acids) are specific fats formed when liquid oils are made into solid fats like shortening and hard margarine. However, a small amount of trans fat is found naturally, primarily in certain animal-based foods.

It may be that the worst ingredients in our food supply are man-altered fats, like hydrogenated oil, partially hydrogenated oil and other trans fats. These oils are very difficult for our bodies to process, and create inflammation throughout the body. Hydrogenated oils make brittle cell walls that do not allow the right nutrients in or the right waste products out. These ingredients are in thousands of food products.

Where Can You Find Trans Fats?

You can find trans fats in almost all boxed items, processed foods, commercial breads, frozen dinners, salad dressings and margarines, cookies, snack foods, crackers, fried foods, baked goods and other foods made with or fried in partially hydrogenated oils. Trans fats behave like saturated fat by raising low-density lipoprotein (LDL or "bad") cholesterol that increases your risk of coronary heart disease. Trans fats are used because they increase the shelf life and flavor stability of foods.

As of January 1, 2006, the Nutrition Facts Labels on packaged food products required by the FDA must include how many grams of trans fatty acid "trans fats" are contained within one serving of the product. The American Heart Association commends the FDA for taking this important step but feels more work is needed to inform consumers about products that do and do not contain trans fats. The American Heart Association recommends a dietary pattern that keeps intake of trans fats and saturated fats as low as possible (with less than ten percent of daily calories coming from trans fats and saturated fats combined) as both of these are associated with an increased risk of heart disease. According to Robert H. Eckel, M.D., president of the American Heart Association and professor of medicine at the University of Colorado at Denver, "Adding trans-fat information to Nutrition Facts Labels on packaged foods is a good start toward providing consumers with the information they need to make informed heart-healthy food choices. Still, consumers should be aware that just because they don't see trans fats on a product label it doesn't necessarily mean that the product is trans fat-free. For example, products with less than 0.5 grams of trans fats can still claim 'zero grams of trans fat' on their label. So just like with 'fat-free' foods, multiple servings of 'zero trans fat' and 'zero saturated fat' products can actually add up to more than 10 percent of daily calories. Also, trans fats and saturated fats can be lurking in places that do not require labeling, like restaurants and cafeterias. We need to continue to expand consumer access to this information in all of these locations so consumers can make healthy decisions in all situations."

Good Fats

Pure, extra-virgin olive oil is not only a light and delicate addition to many wonderful meals, it is one of the most health-promoting types of oils available. Olive oil is rich in monounsaturated fats, a type of fat that researchers are discovering has excellent health benefits.

Studies on olive oil and atherosclerosis reveal that particles of LDL cholesterol (the potentially harmful cholesterol) that contain the monounsaturated fats of olive oil are less likely to become oxidized. Since only oxidized cholesterol sticks to artery walls, eventually forming the plaques that can lead to a heart attack or stroke, preventing the oxidation of cholesterol is a good way to help prevent atherosclerosis.

Coconut oil has a unique role in the diet as an important physiologically functional food. The health and nutritional benefits that can be derived from consuming coconut oil have been recognized in many parts of the world for centuries. A review of the diet/heart disease literature relevant to coconut oil clearly indicates that coconut oil is at worst neutral with respect to atherogenicity of fats and oils and, in fact, is likely to be a beneficial oil for prevention and treatment of some heart disease.

Other oils low in saturated fats and trans fats are corn oil, safflower oil, sunflower oil, soy oil or canola oil. These oils have higher smoke points which make them better to use for fried foods.

Canola, olive, peanut, high oleic safflower and sunflower oils, and nuts are rich in monounsaturated fats. Sources of alpha-linolenic and linoleic acids, which are unsaturated fats and essential oils, include vegetable oils, walnuts, and flaxseed.

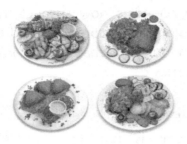

CHAPTER 5

MEAT, POULTRY, FISH DEPARTMENT

Where's The Beef?

Think about all those recipes that include beef, pork, or poultry. This list can be never-ending. So, how concerned should we be with consuming these products? What are we actually digesting in our bodies? This chapter is designed to clarify these questions and many more about the quality of meat, fish, and poultry at your grocery store.

Our grandparents rarely heard of autoimmune diseases. Wikipedia states "Autoimmunity is the failure of an organism to recognize its own constituent parts (down to the sub-molecular levels) as "self" which results in an immune response against its own cells and tissues. Any disease that results from such an abnormal immune response is termed an autoimmune disease. Prominent examples include: heart disease, fibromyalgia, asthma, allergies, irritable bowel syndrome, osteoporosis, degenerative joint disease, inflammation, Celiac disease, diabetes mellitus type 1, systemic lupus erythematosus, Sjögren's syndrome, multiple sclerosis, Hashimoto's thyroiditis, Graves' disease, and rheumatoid arthritis. There are many more.

Some medical scientists now suspect that the increasing occurrence of autoimmune disorders is tied to the widespread use of hormones in food. This chapter explains where hormones are used and what they do.

What are Hormones?

Hormones are chemicals that are produced naturally in the bodies of all animals, including humans. They release chemical messages into the blood via hormone-producing organs; these chemical messages are sent to all parts of the body. Hormones are produced usually in small amounts. They control important body functions such as growth, development and reproduction. Hormones can have different chemical makeups. They can be steroids or proteins. Steroid hormones are active in the body when eaten. For example, birth control pills are steroid hormones and can be taken orally. Protein hormones are broken down in the stomach, and lose their ability to act in the body when eaten. Therefore, protein hormones need to be injected into the body to have an effect. For example, insulin is a protein hormone. Diabetic patients need to be injected with insulin for treatment.

Why are Hormones Used in Food Production?

Certain hormones can make young animals gain weight faster. In dairy cows, hormones can be used to increase milk production. Thus, hormones can increase the profitability of the meat and dairy industries. Why should we be concerned about hormones in foods? While a variety of hormones are produced by our bodies and are essential for normal development of healthy tissue, synthetic steroid hormones used as pharmaceutical drugs have been found to be a risk for causing cancer. For example, diethylstilbestrol (DES), a synthetic estrogen used in the 1960s was withdrawn from use after it was found to increase the risk of vaginal cancer in daughters of women who had used this drug.

What is the relationship? Consumers are increasingly concerned about whether they are being exposed to hormones used to treat animals, and whether these hormones affect human health. This is a complicated issue that can be addressed with the scientific evidence that is currently available via the internet.

History of Hormone use in Food Production

As early as the 1930s, it was realized that cows injected with material drawn from bovine (cow) pituitary glands (hormone secreting organ) produced more milk. Later, the bovine growth hormone (bGH) from the pituitary glands was found to be responsible for this effect. Technology could not harvest enough of this material for large scale use in animals. In the 1980s, it became possible to produce large quantities of pure bGH by using recombinant DNA technology. In 1993, the FDA approved the recombinant bovine growth hormone (rBGH), also known as bovine somatotropin (rbST), for use in dairy cattle. Recent estimates by the manufacturer of this hormone indicate a large percentage of the cows in the United States may be treated with rBGH.

The female sex hormone estrogen was also shown to affect growth rates in cattle and poultry in the 1930s. Once the chemistry of estrogen was understood, it became possible to make the hormone synthetically in large amounts. Synthetic estrogen was used to increase the size of cattle and chickens in the early 1950s. DES was one of the first synthetic estrogens made and used commercially in the US to fatten chickens. It was also used as a drug in human medicine. DES was subsequently found to cause cancer and its use in food production was phased out in the late 1970s.

Artificial Hormones

In 2005, 32.5 million cattle were slaughtered to provide beef for US consumers. Scientists believe about two thirds of American cattle raised for slaughter is injected with hormones to make them grow faster. America's dairy cows are also given a rBGH to increase milk production. These measures mean higher profits for the beef and dairy industries, but what does it mean for consumers? Although the USDA and FDA claim these hormones are safe, there is growing concern that hormone residues in meat and milk might be harmful to human health.

What's in the Beef?

According to the European Union's Scientific Committee on Veterinary Measures Relating to Public Health, the use of six natural and artificial growth hormones in beef pose a potential risk to human health. These six hormones include three which are naturally occurring: estradiol, progesterone and testosterone, and three which are synthetic: zeranol, trenbolone, and melengestrol. The Committee also questioned whether hormone residue in the meat of "growth enhanced" animals can disrupt human hormone balance, cause developmental problems, interfere with the reproductive system, and even lead to the development of breast, prostate or colon cancer. Children, pregnant women and the unborn are thought to be most susceptible to these negative health effects. Hormone residues in beef have been implicated in the early onset of puberty in girls, which could put them at greater risk of developing breast and other forms of cancer. The European Union's Committee reported that as of 1999, no comprehensive studies had been conducted to determine whether hormone residues in meat might be cancer causing. Scientists are also concerned about the environmental impacts of hormone residue in cow manure. Growth-promoting hormones not only remain in the meat we consume, but they pass through the cattle and are excreted in their manure. When manure from factory farms enters the surrounding environment, these hormones can contaminate surface and groundwater. Aquatic ecosystems are particularly vulnerable to hormone residues. Recent studies have demonstrated that exposure to hormones has a substantial effect on the gender and reproductive capacity of fish, throwing off the natural cycle. Despite international scientific concern, the

United States and Canada continue to allow growth promoting hormones in cattle. The European Union, however, does not allow the use of hormones in cattle production, has prohibited the import of hormone-treated beef since 1988, and has banned all beef imports from the U.S. The ban has been challenged by the U.S. at the World Trade Organization and debate still rages between the U.S. and the E.U. over the safety of rBGH.

Antibiotics and Growth Hormones in Feed Lots

Antibiotics and growth hormones are increasingly used in feedlots. Antibiotics are used in feed as well as in injections, vitamins, vaccinations, and parasite controls. Antibiotics are generally administered off and on for 90 days or more in feedlots in the United States. Animals arriving in feedlots are given antibiotics in their water for 8 days or so. Most cattle in U.S. feedlots are given growth hormones to maximize their weight gain. In short, there is significant use of antibiotics, vaccinations, growth hormones, and vitamins in the beef industry and the administration has little understanding of their overall impact.

Harmful Impacts

It is well known that the prophylactic use of antibiotics can lead to bacterial resistance in the animals and in the environment, and that this resistance can even be passed on to bacteria that infect humans. Antibiotics not only kill off the bad bacteria, but also kill off the good or friendly bacteria that humans need to maintain immune system health. Similarly, the effects of growth hormones in the production of meat may be passed on to people who consume the meat (Program on Breast Cancer and Environmental Risk Factors in New York State, 2000). Unfortunately, little research has been undertaken on the impact of antibiotics. Since 1989 Europe has banned the import of US and Canadian beef produced with growth hormones such as estradiol, a potent cancer-causing estrogen. These beef hormones are implanted in pellet form under the skin in the ear of cattle to force them to grow faster, proportionate to increasing industry profits by approximately $80 per animal. Most US beef (90% of all feedlot cattle according to the Cattlemen's Beef Association) is now hormone implanted. Yet lab rats fed these hormones have developed cancer, and at least three of the most commonly used beef hormones appear on state and federal lists as "known" carcinogens. The FDA and USDA (US Department of Agriculture) insist, however, that these beef hormones are totally safe, and that hormone tainted beef need not be labeled. The USDA claims beef hormone residues pose no danger, but then admit they don't test for them except on rare occasions. As a result few American beef eaters know if they're likely getting an extra dose of hormones and estrogen with their burger or steak.

Do Federal Agencies Monitor for The Presence Of These Hormones in Food?

Estradiol, progesterone and testosterone are sex hormones that are made naturally by animals. No regulatory monitoring of these hormones is possible, since it is not possible to separate or tell the difference between the hormones used for treatment from those made by the animal's own body. However, it is possible to detect residues of zeranol and trembolone acetate in the animal's meat. The FDA has set tolerance levels for these hormones. A tolerance is the maximum amount of a particular residue that may be permitted in or on food (see BCERF Fact Sheet #25 on Pesticide Residue Monitoring and Food Safety). The Food Safety Inspection Service (FSIS) of the USDA monitors meat from cattle for zeranol residues. FSIS also monitors meats for DES residues from any illegal use since DES use is no longer permitted. In response to concern about cases of early puberty in Puerto Rico described below, a large number of meat samples were tested for hormone residues in the mid to late 1980s. No zeranol or DES residues were found in the meat samples in this survey.

Can Steroid Hormones in Meat Affect The Age Of Puberty for Girls?

Early puberty in girls has been found to be associated with a higher risk for breast cancer (see CERF Fact Sheet #08, Childhood Life Events and the Risk of Breast Cancer). The exposure to higher than normal levels of steroid hormones though treated beef or poultry has never been documented. Large epidemiological studies have not been done to see whether or not early puberty in developing girls is associated with having eaten growth hormone treated foods. Concerns about an increase in cases of girls reaching puberty or menarche at age eight or younger in Puerto Rico led to an investigation in the early 1980s by the Centers for Disease Control (CDC). Samples of meat and chicken from Puerto Rico were tested for steroid hormone residues. One laboratory found a chicken sample from a local market to have higher than normal level of estrogen. Also, residues of zeranol were reported in the blood of some of the girls who had reached puberty early. However, these results could not be verified by other laboratories. Following the CDC's investigation, the USDA tested 150 to 200 beef, poultry and milk samples from Puerto Rico in 1985 and found no residues of DES, zeranol or estrogen in these samples. In another study in Italy, steroid hormone residues in beef and poultry in school meals were suspected as the cause of breast enlargement in very young girls and boys. However, the suspect beef and poultry samples were not available to test for the presence of hormones. Without proof that exposure to higher levels of steroid hormones occurred through food, it's not possible to conclude whether or not eating hormone treated meat or poultry caused the breast enlargement in these cases.

Can Eating Meat from Hormone Treated Animals Affect Risk for Breast Cancer?

Evidence does not exist to answer this question. The amount of steroid hormone that is eaten through meat of a treated animal is negligible compared to what the human body produces each day. The breast cancer risk in women who eat meat from hormone treated animals has not been compared with the risk of women who eat meat from untreated animals.

Does the E.coli Risk Decrease with Grass Fed Beef?

Grass fed beef has a minimal risk compared to grain fed beef due to the difference in influence on stomach pH between the two diets. Grain diets create a much higher level of acidity in the stomach, which the E.coli bacteria need to survive. Grass fed animals live in grass pastures where higher levels of sanitation greatly reduce the risk of infection as well.

Are Hormone Treated Animals Healthy?

There is a concern that because of increased milking, hormone treated cows may become more prone to infection of the udders, called mastitis. This could lead to more antibiotics being used to treat the cows, in turn leading to more antibiotic residues in milk. Frequent exposure to antibiotic residues through milk or dairy products could be a health concern for people. In the normal body, your good bacteria are found living in your saliva and help throughout your whole digestive tract. These good bacteria help with the digestion of food. They are referred to as "friendly" bacteria and do not generate disease since the immune system keeps them in check. However, if the immune system is weak, these "friendly" bacteria can be overcome by infectious bacteria, thereby developing infection. Infectious bacteria can then frequently develop ways to survive the antibiotics and become "antibiotic resistant." In cases of infection and illness, it then becomes more difficult to control resistant bacteria with antibiotics. Some increase in incidence of antibiotic residues was observed in cow's milk following the use of rBGH. At the same time as rBGH started being used, some of the major dairy states in US switched over to a new and improved method to test for antibiotic residues. It is difficult to determine whether the increase in incidence of antibiotic residues in milk was due to increased use or to better testing methods. New York State was one of the states that had not changed its method to test for antibiotic residues in milk at that time. The incidence of antibiotic residues in milk from New York State was not found to be higher. This suggests that the increased incidence of antibiotic residues observed in some states may have been due to better testing methods rather than an increase in use of antibiotics. An Expert Committee at FDA's Center for Veterinary Medicine has concluded that while the overuse of antibiotics may cause a slight increase in mastitis, dairy management practices that are currently in use should prevent any increase in antibiotic residues in milk.

What is CLA?

CLA (conjugated linoleic acid) is a fatty acid mixture found in nature, which does not have any known negative side effects. The most abundant source of natural CLA is in the meat and dairy products of grass fed animals. Research conducted since 1999 shows that grazing animals have from three to five times more CLA than animals fattened on grain in a feedlot. Simply switching from grain fed to grass fed products can greatly increase your intake of CLA. There is a reason why it may be beneficial to allow cows to graze on pasture, and it involves a CLA in beef and dairy fats. University of Wisconsin scientists researched and discovered in a study of rats that ate grass fed hamburger, the CLA constitution has cancer-fighting properties. CLA cannot be produced by the human body, but it can be obtained through foods such as whole milk, butter, beef, and lamb. "The interesting thing is that dairy cattle that graze produce higher amounts of CLA in their milk than those which receive conserved feed, such as grain, hay, and silage," says ARS dairy scientist Larry Satter. "This is true even when the non-grazers eat pasture grass conserved as hay." Satter, based at the Dairy Forage Research Center in Madison, Wisconsin, conducted a study comparing the amount of CLA in milk from cows grazing on pasture to the amount from cows fed hay or silage. His findings: pasture-grazed cows had five times more CLA in their milk than those fed silage. Grass fed organic production protocol ensures that the quality of the product you receive is consistent time after time. Here is what you can count on. Grass fed beef is not irradiated. No hormonal growth implants are used to speed up growth and weight gain. No feed grade antibiotics are used. Grass diets eliminate this concern and risk, so no unnecessary antibiotics are used. Just like humans, animals sometimes become ill and need antibiotics. Should this occur, meat producers record and track the injection. The animal must then meet protocol for "double the industry standard" withdrawal time from the medication, prior to processing. Animal by-products are also used by some feedlots as cost saving feed ingredients. These are taboo for grass fed beef products.

Why Use Feedlot Cows?

Cows raised in feedlots are ready for market seven months faster than grass fed cows. The key to profit in the grain or corn fed beef industry, which operates on extremely low individual margin, is volume and speed. The sooner an animal can be brought to slaughter, the higher the volume and hence the greater the profit in the grocery store beef industry. Once placed in a feedlot, hyped up on growth hormones and grain or corn fed, the animal can be pushed to gains of 3.5 to 5 pounds a day.

Eight Major Factors for the Higher Cost of Grass Fed Beef

1. Additional land is required for grass fed beef.
2. Quality of the land has to be higher.
3. Veterinarian owner overseeing the cattle must establish precise protocols for farming methods.
4. Time to bring the cattle to market is longer (average seven months longer).
5. Labor is involved to assure that the cattle receive optimal care, low stress and excellent nutrition.

MEAT, POULTRY, FISH DEPARTMENT

6. Butcher processing uses dry aging rather than unskilled mass production methods with no aging.
7. Economies of scale for a large corporation versus an individual grass farm.
8. Small shipments to individuals rather hundreds of pounds of beef sides and whole beef delivered in semi trucks.

Why the Price Difference When Grass is Free?

Grass fed beef is usually much more expensive than grain fed beef. So why the difference if grass is free? Actually, grass isn't free. In August 2002, the USDA's National Agricultural Statistics Service (NASS) reported, "U.S. farm real estate values, including land in buildings, averaged $1,210 per acre as of January 1, 2002, up over five percent from the previous year." And every year acreage value increases a minimum of five percent.

Antibiotics In Poultry May Pose Risk to Humans

Could a turkey sandwich or a bowl of chicken soup be hazardous to your health? Poultry has that potential, according to research that suggests people who eat drug treated poultry may be at increased risk of developing antibiotic resistance. Still, the findings are preliminary and shouldn't make anyone stop eating chicken or turkey, the study's lead investigator said. "We don't want to suggest to anyone that they should alter their diet based on this," said Dr. Edward Belongia, director of the Marshfield Clinic Research Foundation's Epidemiology Research Center in Wisconsin. "But federal regulators should consider the results as they make rules about the kinds of drugs given to poultry," the investigator added. The issue is the use of virginiamycin, an antibiotic used in farm animals to boost their growth. The drug is banned in Europe, but farmers are allowed to use it in the United States. Some studies have suggested that virginiamycin can cause germs in poultry to become super-powered, like the overuse of antibiotics in humans has made some infectious bacteria immune to certain drugs. This phenomenon, known as drug resistance, happens when an antibiotic is used so often that germs mutate around it. It's also possible for drug resistance to be spread through food. "When we consume food with organisms that have resistant genes, these genes can be transferred to our natural organisms, causing them to become drug-resistant," explained Molly Marten, a clinical epidemiologist at Scripps Mercy Hospital in San Diego familiar with the study findings.

Belongia and colleagues launched their study to see if people who ate chicken or turkey treated with antibiotics would lead to the development of antibiotic-resistant bacteria. They isolated Enterococcus faecium, a gut bacterium that is increasingly the cause of infections in hospitals, in stool samples from 105 newly-hospitalized patients and 65 healthy vegetarians, as well as in 77 samples of conventional retail poultry and 23 antibiotic-free poultry meat samples. After exposure to virginiamycin, E. faecium from conventional poultry and from patients who consumed poultry became resistant to the antibiotic Synercid more often than E. faecium from vegetarians or from antibiotic-free poultry. Some of the resistance was attributed to a specific gene and both the gene and resistance were associated with touching raw poultry meat and frequent poultry consumption. Furthermore, patients who ate the most chicken seemed most susceptible to developing drug resistant bacteria, as did those who touched poultry. "Right now, this isn't a major problem because Synercid isn't used a great deal," Belongia said. "That means germs haven't had a chance to become immune to it. But that could change," he said. Belongia believes that the U.S. Food and Drug Administration should take the findings into account. In a written statement, advised that antibiotics should not be used to promote growth in animals.

Pork, Antibiotics, and Hormones

Over the last 17 years, U.S. pork producers have dramatically decreased the need for antibiotics by lowering disease threats through sound herd management and by using drugs only when needed. The industry introduced the Take Care, Use Antibiotics Responsibly Program in early 2005. This program focuses on raising awareness and guiding producers on the responsible use of antibiotics. The Take Care program has the support of veterinarians, the pharmaceutical industry, and the Centers for Disease Control. Take Care raises the awareness of the public regarding agricultural antibiotic use. The program encourages producers to implement management practices that reduce the need for antibiotics, and to use antibiotics only when other management practices do not, or will not, succeed in managing a correctly diagnosed problem.

Animal Well-Being

U.S. pork producers take pride and personal responsibility in providing proper animal care on their farms. They consider anything short of the best, most humane care as self-defeating. Today's consumer wants to know that pigs have been raised under humane conditions.

The National Pork Board has developed the Swine Welfare Assurance Program (SWAP), a voluntary, science-based program to help pork producers to objectively assess and benchmark the care and welfare of their pigs. The SWAP development panel includes international welfare experts, veterinarians and pork producers. The objective of the program is to maintain and promote the pork industry's tradition of responsible animal care through the application of scientifically sound animal care practices. Since its introduction in 2003, SWAP has been adopted by producers of all sizes and types. U.S. pork production continues to lead agriculture in the adoption of new technologies and has achieved record-high productivity. The increased productivity translates to efficiencies that mean not only that is pork higher quality and safer than at any time in history, but also that it costs 20 percent less than it did in 1979.

Organic Meats, Chicken and Poultry

More and more consumers are wondering if they should be purchasing organic foods, including meat, chicken or fish, due to concerns about consuming foods that may contain antibiotics and growth hormones, questions that arise include:

- Are livestock fed non-genetically engineered feed?
- Are pastures without animal remnants which guard from mad cow?
- Are animals treated humanely (for example: open space, no cage)?

Organic Beef, Pork, or Poultry Is Legally Defined As:

Coming from animals that weren't offspring of cloned animals, were raised on 100% organic feed, not given growth hormones, antibiotics or other drugs. Additionally, the meat has not been irradiated. In the U.S., foods must be certified in order for the food to be marketed as organic. When referring to organic vs. natural beef there are apparent differences. Organic has to do with how food is grown (how the animals are raised). Natural, on the other hand, deals with how a food product is processed. Further terms used by the USDA in classifying food are as follows:

- Certified: Implies that the USDA's food safety and inspection service and the agricultural marketing service have officially evaluated a meat product for class grade, or other quality characteristics.
- Free-range or free roaming: Producers must demonstrate to the agency that the poultry has been allowed access to the outside.
- Natural: A product containing no artificial ingredient or added color that is only minimally processed (in a way that does not fundamentally alter the raw product) may be labeled natural. The label must explain the use of the term natural (such as no added colorings or artificial ingredients: minimally processed).

- No hormones: Hormones are not allowed in raising hogs or poultry. Therefore, the claim "no hormones added" cannot be used on the labels of pork or poultry unless it is followed by a statement that says, "Federal regulations prohibit the use of hormones ."
- No hormones (beef): The phrase "no hormones administered" may be approved for use on the label of beef products if sufficient documentation is provided to the agency by the producer showing no hormones have been used in raising the animals.
- No antibiotics (red meat or poultry): The phrase "no antibiotics added" may be used on labels for meat or poultry products if sufficient documentation is provided by the producer to the agency demonstrating that the animals were raised without antibiotics. All certified organic meat is independently inspected and monitored at every phase of production to ensure compliance with USDA National Organic Standards.

Organic vs. Non-Organic

When animals are 100% grass-fed, their meat is not only lower in saturated fats but also slightly higher in omega-3 fatty acids. This healthy fat is the same fat found in salmon and flaxseed, which studies indicate reduces disease, including the risk for heart disease, and bolsters the immune system. Dr. Steve Atchley, an advocate for health conscious meat says, "Any feedlot-fattened animal has a much higher level of saturated fat than a forage-fed steer." Furthermore, grass fed beef is lower in calories and, as mentioned before, contains more CLA, which recent studies suggest may decrease the risk for breast cancer, diabetes and other ailments. In addition, grass-fed meat is higher than grain-finished meat in vitamins A and E.

One ranching practice that has become a serious health problem is the grain-based diet offered to cattle. A grain diet breeds an acid resistant form of E. coli in cattle which can be transmitted by feces and dead carcasses. Overuse of antibiotics in grain-based cattle diets has also caused resistance among many types of bacteria.

Is Organic Beef Healthier?

Based on the fact that organic meats are free of many antibiotics and hormones, organics also tend to have fewer pesticides as well. Evidence also suggests that grass fed beef may be healthier than beef raised in traditional feedlots. Generally, grass fed cattle are slaughtered at smaller weights than grain fed beef, producing leaner cuts of beef and a lower percentage of fat.

Where is More Research Needed?

What is a safe and healthier way of eating meat? Based on conservative estimates, the amount of estradiol in two hamburgers eaten by an eight-year-old boy could increase his hormone levels by 10%. Much higher hormone levels are found in meat products following illegal implantation in cattle muscle tissue, which is commonplace in U.S. feedlots. A random survey of 32 large feedlots found that as many as half of the cattle had visible "misplaced implants" in muscle, rather than under ear skin. Lifelong exposure to high residues of natural and synthetic sex hormones in meat products poses serious risks for breast and reproductive cancers, which have sharply increased in the US since 1950. Hormone residues are also suspected to be causal factors in premature sexual development in young girls.

Some of the consumer concerns cannot be answered conclusively without further studies. Exposure to hormones in meat was suspected as the cause for early puberty in girls in Puerto Rico and Italy, but was never verified. Large scale studies would be needed to compare the age of puberty in girls who eat meat from hormone treated animals to those who eat meat from untreated animals. Such studies would need to make sure that other known influences that affect the age of puberty in girls are not playing a role. Short term studies in laboratory rats have not indicated a concern about milk-related allergies or immune effects from exposure to rBGH or IGF-1 in milk or dairy products. However, short term studies cannot rule out the possibility of any immune or unexpected health effects after long term exposure. Studies in laboratory animals on the effects of life-long exposure to milk from rBGH treated cows may help answer this question. By following some healthy diet tips you can help reduce exposure to hormones used in food production. While currently available evidence does not indicate a link between eating meat, milk or dairy products from hormone treated animals and negative health effects, adopting some known healthy habits can reduce your exposure to hormones used in meat, poultry and dairy production.

Wild Salmon vs. Farm Raised Salmon

In January 2001, BBC News produced the program, "Warnings from the Wild, The Price of Salmon," a program pilot study conducted by a Dr. Michael Easton of the David Suzuki Foundation. The study found that farm raised salmon and the feed they ate appeared to have a much higher level of contamination with respect to PCBs (polychlorinated biphenyls) and PBDEs (polybrominated diphenyl ethers) than did wild salmon. It concluded that some contamination in farmed fish comes from the feed.

In July 2003, the Environmental Working Group, EWG, released a report stating that farm raised salmon purchased in the United States contains the highest level of PCBs in the food supply system. In the report, EWG reported that farm raised salmon has 16 times the amount of PCBs found in wild salmon, three to four times the levels found in other seafood, and four times the levels found in beef. EWG recommends that consumers choose wild salmon instead of farm raised salmon, and that they should eat an eight ounce serving of farm raised salmon no more than once a month.

In January 2004, the journal Science warned that farm raised salmon contains ten times more toxins (PCBs, dioxin, etc.) than wild salmon. The study recommends that farm raised salmon be eaten no more than once a month, or perhaps no more than every two months as it poses cancer risks to human beings.

Why Do Farm Raised Salmon Contain More PCBs than Wild Salmon?

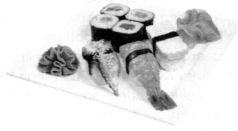

Studies found that the fishmeal fed to farm raised salmon is highly contaminated with PCBs. Farm raised salmon are fatter, and they are generally bigger in size and contain more fat than wild salmon. PCBs are stored in fat and remain there for an extended period of time; therefore farm raised salmon contains more PCBs.

Government Guidelines

The average level of PCBs in salmon is 0.027 ppm (parts per million).

- FDA: The current FDA limit of PCBs in all fish is 2 ppm.
- Health Canada: The current guideline for PCBs in fish is 2 ppm.
- EPA: The current recommendation is between 0.024 and 0.048 ppm

The Environmental Protection Agency guideline on PCBs is much stricter. They recommend that fish with PCB levels between 0.024 to 0.048 ppm should be restricted to no more than eight ounces a month.

What Does This All Mean?

There is an obvious discrepancy in the limits set by various health agencies. Dr. Mark Woodin of Tufts University noted that even if the strict EPA guidelines were known to be the right ones, they are based on the amount of PCBs that are thought to be capable of causing one additional cancer case in 100,000 people over a 70-year lifetime.

Key Message

Don't give up fish and salmon completely. It is a known fact that fish and salmon offer benefits in heart health. The benefits may outweigh the risk of getting cancer from eating farmed salmon. Choose a variety of fish and include them in a healthy well-balanced diet and practice the following: trim the skin and the fat as PCBs are stored in the fat portion. Prepare your salmon to reduce the fat by using techniques such as grilling and broiling. Try canned salmon since almost all types of this salmon is wild.

What You Need To Know About Mercury in Fish and Shellfish

For women who might become pregnant, women who are pregnant, nursing mothers, and young children: Fish and shellfish are an important part of a healthy diet. Fish and shellfish contain high-quality protein and other essential nutrients, are low in saturated fat, and contain omega-3 fatty acids. A well-balanced diet that includes a variety of fish and shellfish can contribute to heart health and children's proper growth and development. So, women and young children in particular should include fish or shellfish in their diets due to the many nutritional benefits.

However, nearly all fish and shellfish contain traces of mercury. For most people, the risk from mercury by eating fish and shellfish is not a health concern. Yet, some fish and shellfish contain levels of mercury that may harm an unborn baby or young child's developing nervous system. The risks from mercury in fish and shellfish depend on the amount of fish and shellfish eaten and the levels of mercury in the fish and shellfish. Therefore, the Food and Drug Administration and the Environmental Protection Agency are advising women who may become pregnant, pregnant women, nursing mothers, and young children to avoid some types of fish and eat fish and shellfish that are lower in mercury. By following these three recommendations for selecting and eating fish or shellfish, women and young children will receive the benefits of eating fish and shellfish and be confident that they have reduced their exposure to the harmful effects of mercury: Do not eat Shark, Swordfish, King Mackerel, or Tilefish because they contain high levels of mercury.

- Eat up to 12 ounces (2 average meals) a week of a variety of fish and shellfish that are lower in mercury.
- Five of the most commonly eaten fish that are low in mercury are shrimp, canned light tuna, salmon, pollock, and catfish.
- Another commonly eaten fish, albacore ("white") tuna has more mercury than canned light tuna. So, when choosing your two meals of fish and shellfish, you may eat up to 6 ounces (one average meal) of albacore tuna per week. Check local advisories about the safety of fish caught by family and friends in your local lakes, rivers, and coastal areas. If no advice is available, eat up to 6 ounces (one average meal) per week of fish you catch from local waters, but don't consume any other fish during that week.

Follow these same recommendations when feeding fish and shellfish to your young child, but serve smaller portions.

Frequently Asked Questions about Mercury in Fish and Shellfish:

"What are mercury and methylmercury?"
Mercury occurs naturally in the environment and can also be released into the air through industrial pollution. Mercury falls from the air and can accumulate in streams and oceans and is then turned into methylmercury in the water. It is this type of mercury that can be harmful to your unborn baby and young child. Fish absorb the methylmercury as they feed in these waters

and so it builds up in them. It builds up more in some types of fish and shellfish than others, depending in what the fish eat.

"Should a woman who is not pregnant, but planning to become pregnant be concerned about methylmercury?"
If you regularly eat types of fish that are high in methylmercury, it can accumulate in your bloodstream over time. Methylmercury is removed from the body naturally, but it may take over a year for the levels to drop significantly. Thus, it may be present in a woman even before she becomes pregnant. This is the reason why women who are trying to become pregnant should also avoid eating certain types of fish.

"Is there methylmercury in all fish and shellfish?"
Nearly all fish and shellfish contain traces of methylmercury. However, larger fish that have lived longer have the highest levels of methylmercury because they've had more time to accumulate it. These large fish (swordfish, shark, king mackerel and tilefish) pose the greatest risk. Other types of fish and shellfish may be eaten in the amounts recommended by FDA and EPA.

"I don't see the fish I eat in the advisory, what should I do?"
If you want more information about the levels in the various types of fish you eat, see the FDA food safety website: www.cfsan.fda.gov/frf/sea-mehg.html, or the EPA website at www.epa.gov/ost/fish.

"What about fish sticks and fast food sandwiches?"
Fish sticks and "fast-food" sandwiches are commonly made from fish that are low in mercury.

"The advice about canned tuna is a great recommendation, but what's the advice about tuna steaks?"
Because tuna steak generally contains higher levels of mercury than canned light tuna, when choosing your two meals of fish

and shellfish, you may eat up to 6 ounces (one average meal) of tuna steak per week.

"What if I eat more than the recommended amount of fish and shellfish in a week?"
One week's consumption of fish does not change the level of methylmercury in the body much at all. If you eat a lot of fish one week, you can cut back for the next week or two. Just make sure you average the recommended amount per week.

"Where do I get information about the safety of fish caught recreationally by family or friends?"
Before you go fishing, check your Fishing Regulations Booklet for information about recreationally caught fish. You can also contact your local health department for information about local advisories. You need to check local advisories because some kinds of fish and shellfish caught in your local waters may have higher or much lower than average levels of mercury. This depends on the levels of mercury in the water where the fish are caught. Those fish with much lower levels may be eaten more frequently and in larger amounts.

    For further information about the risks of mercury in fish and shellfish call the U.S. Food and Drug Administration's food information line toll-free at 1-888-SAFEFOOD or visit federal Food Safety website: http://www.foodsafety.gov/

    For further information about the safety of locally caught fish and shellfish, visit the Environmental Protection Agency's Fish Advisory website: www.epa.gov/ost/fish or contact your State or Local Health Department.

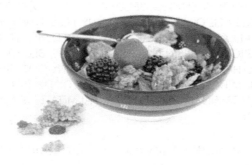

CHAPER 6
CEREAL AISLE

Sugar Cereal Breakfast

Unfortunately, Fruity Pebbles is not really a fruit, nor does it have any fruit in the cereal. It's not even a cornerstone in the Food Pyramid. A bowl of Apple Jacks cereal a day doesn't keep the doctor away, or the dentist for that matter. After all, a sugar-laced box of cereal is the only way to ensure noblemen such as Cap'n Crunch, Count Chocula, and King Vitamin a place in the family grocery cart. Or you can go right for the hard core Sugar Smacks or Sugar Crisp. Buying a toy or prize inside cereal boxes is a good way to add to home collections. How about the leprechaun who sprinkles sugar on Lucky Charms? I am sure the struggle from sugary cereal to "no sugar added" can be a bitter battle at times, just as other parent-to-child confrontations can be. Read the following cereal ingredients and you will be surprised in what you consume.

Ingredients: RICE, SUGAR, POLYDEXTROSE (SOURCE OF FIBER), HYDROGENATED VEGETABLE OIL (COCONUT AND PALM KERNEL OILS),SALT, CONTAINS LESS THAN 0.5% OF NATURAL AND ARTIFICIAL FLAVOR, RED 40, YELLOW 6, TURMERIC OLEORESIN (COLOR), YELLOW 5, BLUE 1, BLUE 2, BHA (TO HELP PROTECT FLAVOR). VITAMINS AND MINERALS: NIACINAMIDE, REDUCED IRON, ZINC OXIDE (SOURCE OF ZINC), VITAMIN B6, VITAMIN A PALMITATE, RIBOFLAVIN, VITAMIN D.

This is the ingredient listing for Fruit Loops. Doesn't it look nutritious? In case you didn't notice, it contains sugar as the second most abundant ingredient, plus trans fats (hydrogenated vegetable oil), unknown artificial flavor, five separate artificial food colors (red 40, yellow 6, yellow 5, blue 1, and blue 2), and an artificial preservative (BHA). In addition, the phrase "natural and artificial flavor" is meaningless, since federal regulations allow synthetic chemicals to be classified as natural. All the flavors might be artificial!

The impact of high sugar cereals on health is not only from the direct affects of sugar on health. A recent study confirms that young children consuming sugar-sweetened cereal and soda, as opposed to consuming natural food sweetened with fruit, tend to eat less food with a higher nutritional value. Sugar consumption adds poor nutrition and leads to taking in less nutrition from other foods. This is a big double whammy against children's health.

Healthy Breakfast Cereal Overview

Confused at the breakfast cereal aisle? You are not alone. The cereal aisle is changing. You can be overwhelmed by the endless rows of colored boxes on tightly packed shelves. Take a closer look and you will see the numerous health claims and health related logos found on the boxes.

Cereals with Heart Health Claims

Breakfast cereals claim to "help reduce the risk of heart disease" and yes, they possibly can. These claims are approved by the FDA as these cereals contain certain heart-healthy ingredients such as whole grains, psyllium and oats. They usually are low in fat and high in fiber. The only problem is that the ingredients show no recommended percentages of fiber, vitamins or other nutrients to help you assess your daily needs. To obtain the recommended daily value you need to consume the equivalent of eight bowls a day of hot or cold cereal. But wait, if you do that you also consume eight times the food dyes, trans fats, salt, and other ingredients cereal manufacture's like to include in their boxes of cereal.

Cereals containing 100% wheat bran, oat bran and barley have a better nutritional value, and you will feel full longer. Unlike refined corn or rice cereals, these are not rapidly digested and absorbed; therefore, after eating these particular kinds of cereals, you will be less likely to prowl around for pre-lunch snacks.

Cereals with Fruit

Some cereals have added real freeze-dried berries, apples and bananas. However, fruits are usually added in low-fiber, refined-grain cereals. It is a better option to toss in your own fresh fruits. The combination of fresh fruit with cereal provides a better way to lure your children away from sugar-loaded frosted cereals.

Cereals with a Weight Loss Claim

Weight claims seem to be appealing, but are actually fancy marketing tools. Quite a few brands of cereal are found with claims to help you lose weight. These cereals are often low in fat, but the majority of breakfast cereals are low in fat anyway. There is really nothing special about them.

Kellogg's Special K, for instance, has only one gram of fiber per serving. For more waistline-friendly cereal, you might want to choose high fiber, whole grain product.

Cereals with Novel Ingredients

Read the label please! It is not difficult to find cereals that add other ingredients such as pecans, almonds or flaxseeds. Some cereals are even made with soy. Since there are so many varieties, it is best to read the nutrition facts labels. Compare products, and look for the fiber content as well as the sugar content.

Are Reduced-Sugar Cereals Worth It?

A few years ago letters were sent to major cereal manufacturers from conscientious parents or guilt-ridden ones to make the cereals with half the sugar. Kelloggs, General Mills and Post Cereals responded by reformulating a few popular sweetened brands two basic ways. They cut back on the amount of sugar per serving, and began using sucralose (Splenda, a sugar substitute). The new boxes display the words "reduced sugar." You can find new counterparts located near their original versions. Nevertheless, the public has not bought into these low-sugar version completely. A.C. Nielsen data show that, within the one year time period ending October 2004, sales of cereals with less sugar dropped significantly. How many parents are really concerned with the nutrition facts?

What is in the Reduced-Sugar Cereals?

Kelloggs found that the taste and texture of its reduced-sugar Frosted Flakes and Fruit Loops could be maintained with one third the sugar, along with fillers and binders that count as added carbohydrates. General Mills used 75% less sugar in their reduced sugar versions of Cinnamon Toast Crunch, Trix and Cocoa Puffs by adding Splenda. The reduced sugar version of Fruity Pebbles by Post Cereals contains half as much sugar as the standard version. The loss of sweetness was made up by adding sucralose (Splenda) and additional carbohydrates for taste. While new cereal versions succeed in cutting back on sugar, they do not come with benefits of fewer calories (check the side label for the nutritional details).

Reduced-sugar cereals also do not come cheaply. The cereals cost more per ounce than their original versions. Watchful shoppers will notice that original and reduced-sugar cereals come in the same size boxes, but those boxes can differ in total weight by as much as six ounces. Reduced-sugar cereals usually don't seem to go on sale.

How appealing are the reduced sugar cereals to their target market? Five "Kids Post" readers were given a cereal challenge. University of Maryland nutrition professor Mark A. Kantor was asked to help out. The children were given dry cereal to test. They munched their way through 12 sweetened, ready-to-eat cereals, five examples of original brands and their reduced sugar versions, and two new Kellogg's "lightly sweetened" brands. The cereals were dispensed from plain brown lunch bags. There were no clear favorites among the Frosted Flakes, Cocoa Puffs, Cinnamon Toast Crunch, Trix and Fruity Pebbles. However, half the testers correctly identified five sets of cereals that had less sugar. Two of the children decided that the reduced sugar cereals tasted the same as their originals. The majority of the testers favored the regular sweetened cereals. The comments about the original cereals were, "good, natural, sweet, great, better, and "the bomb." "Two young testers said they preferred the reduced-sugar versions of Cocoa Puffs and Trix, but they noted those samples comparatively lacked crunch and sweetness. Another couple of children described the same cereals as "too fruity" or "too weird."

Kantor, the lone adult member of the panel, said, "The kids are absolutely correct that cereals made with 'real' sugar are better-tasting. Even manufacturers agree that no artificial sweetener tastes exactly like sugar." Kantor went further to say, "Sucralose comes close to sugar because its chemical structure is similar to sugar and it does not leave an aftertaste, like saccharin and acesulfame-K."

The panel also tasted Kellogg's two brand new cereals aimed at the preschool crowd, Tiger Power, whose primary sweetness comes from brown sugar, and Hunny B's, which is made with honey. These cereals have fewer grams of sugar per serving compared to regular sweetened cereals. Most of the testers were not impressed with either product.

Here is an article from a typical father (sugar lover) introducing his daughter to a tasty, scrumptious, not really nutritious cereal. It shows how the sweet taste of a sugar cereal can overcome the nutritional value in a wholesome breakfast.

Garret Leiva from the Grand Traverse Herald writes,

> "Confiscate my World's Greatest Dad coffee mug. I let my child partake in forbidden Fruity Pebbles. Right now, grandmothers everywhere are gritting their teeth. Yes, I fortified our two and a half year old with riboflavin and questionable "essential" vitamins. I've given new meaning to the term Sugar Daddy. When it comes to cereal consumption, Ella is a mommy's girl. However, my wife dishes out fruit, fiber and very little sugar at the breakfast table. While my cravings are less than ravenous, I've been known to indulge my taste buds with the red dye #40 of sugar cereals. So there is a logical reason why Ella ended up at the kitchen table with Fred Flintstone and Barney Rubble. Daddy did the grocery shopping last week. With no other breakfast staples in the cupboard, unless you count a jar of Fluff, Ella had her first bowl of sugared cereal, naturally she ate it up."

Bottom Line:

Breakfast is an important meal to start your day. Studies have shown that athletes who do eat breakfast perform better in competition. Children who eat breakfast are able to concentrate better in class. Adults who eat breakfast are able to control weight better than those who do not eat breakfast. The recommended intake of fiber is 25 to 50 grams per day. Choose breakfast cereals with at least 5 grams of fiber per serving. Many cereals with 100% whole grains have much higher amounts of fiber. When reading nutrition labels, pay attention to the sugar content. Cereals with fruits usually have a higher sugar content because sugar naturally occurs in fruits. However, it is shocking to find some cereals, including those marketed to children, containing 15 to 20 grams of refined sugar per serving. That's disgusting!

What, you don't want to give up your favorite frosted cereal? Try mixing and matching! Mix some high fiber whole-grain cereal as well as fresh fruit with sugar cereal. Any steps toward reducing sugar and increasing fiber in your cereal bowl are positive ones!

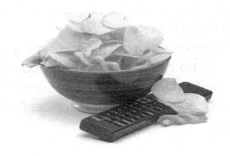

CHAPTER 7
SNACKS, CHIPS, AND CRACKER AISLE

Before I comment the on good and bad snacks, I would like to share some information and history about the ingredients used to make these products. Information about these ingredients will help you decide which ones are best for your health.

Carbohydrates

In the 1990s, low-fat dieting fads resulted in high carbohydrate diets due to overabundance of snacks that advertised their low or no-fat ingredients. Unfortunately, these fats were frequently replaced by sugar and starch and America's weight kept increasing. The continued increase of our waistlines caused us to search for an alternative and the "low carbohydrate, high protein" diet craze began in the early 2000s with the discovery of the Atkins diet. In his clinic, Dr. Robert Atkins utilized an extremely low carbohydrate diet, which was followed systematically until a healthy weight was achieved. At that point, a small amount of carbohydrates could be allowed back into the diet.

Other diet theories, such as those using a glycemic index, claim that some carbohydrates affect the body differently from others. Starchy and sugary foods trigger insulin and glucose (blood sugar) to rise quickly, while higher-fiber foods have a lower impact on glucose.

What is a Carbohydrate?

What carbohydrates (carbs) are good? What carbs are bad? What is a carbohydrate anyway? A carbohydrate is defined at www.Dictionary.com as: "Any of a group of organic compounds that includes sugars, starches, cellulose, and gums and serves as a major energy source in the diet of animals. These compounds are produced by photosynthesis in plants. Sugars, starches, and cellulose are major energy sources produced by plants." This definition does not distinguish cellulose as an energy source for some animals, but not for humans. Cellulose is an indigestible fiber in our diet. Simple carbohydrates, which are found in fruits and dairy products, are more easily digested by the body. They are also often found in processed, refined foods such as white sugar, pastas, and white bread.

Complex carbohydrates, which take longer for the body to digest, are most commonly found in vegetables (as cellulose). Some examples are whole grain breads, brown rice, and legumes. Foods with unrefined grains, such as brown rice, retain complex carbs. Refined grains, such as white rice, do not retain complex carbs since the refining process removes some of the grain's fiber and nutrients. Eating a serving of whole grain cereal such as oatmeal will fill you up and give you longer lasting energy than a bowl of sugary cereal due to the way the body processes and uses the carbohydrates.

The liver digests carbohydrates by breaking them down into simple sugars, or glucose, which stimulates the production of insulin in the pancreas. Insulin works to get the sugar into the body's cells to be used as energy. In comparison with the digestion of complex carbs, the digestion of simple carbs causes insulin levels spike faster, and the carbs are used up more quickly for energy. This explains why many who turn to a candy bar for a quick supply of energy find that their energy levels crash when the "sugar high" comes to an end. Complex carbohydrates take longer to digest, resulting in longer lasting energy and less of an insulin reaction in the body.

Types of Carbohydrates

There are basically four types of carbohydrates in nutrition: sugars, starches, fibers and gums. Sugars usually make things taste sweet. We find sugar in fruits as fructose, in sugar beets and sugar cane as sucrose, and in milk as lactose. Another type of sugar is glucose, which is the simple form of sugar our bodies use for fuel. Starches are long chains or branched chains of glucose and sometimes other sugars. The starches are used to store energy in plants. Some vegetables, like potatoes and corn have a lot of starch, while others have very little, like green beans and spinach.

Fiber is also found in plants. Fiber is a carbohydrate that our body can't digest, so it passes through the digestive system. You might commonly hear about two types of fiber called soluble and insoluble. Soluble fiber is found in fruits, flax seeds, and oats. Soluble fiber helps to reduce cholesterol, and slows down the absorption of sugar into our blood.

Carbohydrates that are often used as fillers and thickeners are carageenan and guar gum. The guar gum crop usually comes from India and Pakistan. Chewing gum is made from guar gum. Carrageenan comes from algae or seaweed and can be used as a thickening agent in place of animal-based products like gelatin. It is derived from a red alga called Irish moss. Carrageenan is a common ingredient in many foods such as milk products like yogurt.

Crackers-Not all they are Cracked Up to Be

Fat is good. Fat is bad. Fat is in. Fat is out. The swings of the pendulum particularly irk those who need to design products that ideally require a certain measure of fat, and most crackers fall into that category.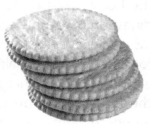

Crackers have been attracting attention as nutritional concerns, prompting manufacturer's to modify recipes. Some have developed crackers high in fiber, others are promoting the low-cholesterol aspect of their brands, while still others have begun marketing low-salt versions of old favorites. But the most widely publicized change has been the substitution of polyunsaturated vegetable fats for highly saturated tropical oils and animal fats.

Despite these changes, many crackers are still high in fat, sodium and calories.

Chips and Their Origin

The popularity of potato chips quickly spread across the country in the early 1900s, particularly in speakeasies, spawning a flurry of home-based companies. Van de Camp's Saratoga Chips opened in Los Angeles on January 6, 1915. In 1921, Earl Wise, a grocer, was stuck with an overstock of potatoes. He peeled them, sliced them with a cabbage cutter and then fried them according to his mother's recipe and packaged them in brown paper bags. Leonard Japp and George Gavora started Jays Foods in the early 1920s, selling potato chips, nuts, and pretzels to speakeasies from the back of a dilapidated truck.

The chips were commonly prepared in someone's kitchen and then delivered immediately to stores and restaurants, or sold on the street. The shelf-life of these chips was virtually nil. Two innovations paved the way for mass production. In 1925, the automatic potato-peeling machine was invented. A year later, several employees at Laura Scudder's potato chip company ironed sheets of waxed paper into bags. The chips were hand-packed into the bags, which were then ironed shut.

Potato chips received a further boost when the U.S. government declared them an essential food in 1942, allowing factories to remain open during World War II. In many cases, potato chips were the only ready-to-eat vegetables available. After the war, it was commonplace to serve chips with dips. French onion soup mix stirred into sour cream was the overall favorite. Television also contributed to the chip's popularity as Americans brought snacks with them when they settled in front of their television sets each night.

In 1969, General Mills and Proctor & Gamble introduced fabricated potato chips, Chipos and Pringles®, respectively. They were made from potatoes that had been cooked, mashed, dehydrated, reconstituted into dough, and cut into uniform pieces. They further differed from previous chips in that they were packaged into break-proof, oxygen-free canisters. The Potato Chip Institute (now the Snack Food Association) filed suit to prevent General Mills and Proctor & Gamble from calling their products chips. Although the suit was dismissed, the USDA did stipulate that the new variety must be labeled as "potato chips made from dried potatoes." Although they are still on the market, fabricated chips have never achieved the popularity of the original.

Today, potato chips are the most popular snack in the United States. According to the Snack Food Association, potato chips constitute 40% of snack food consumption, beating out pretzels and popcorn in spite of the fact that hardly anyone thinks potato chips are nutritious. Nonetheless, the major challenge faced by manufacturers in the 1990s was to develop a tasty low-fat potato chip.

Raw Material

To start the chip making process, potatoes are fried in either corn oil, cottonseed oil, or a blend of vegetable oils. An anti-oxidizing agent is added to the oil to prevent rancidity. To ensure that it stays pure over tome, the oil is passed through a filtration system daily. Some seasonings used to flavor chips are salt, powdered sour cream, onion, and barbecue flavor. Flake salt is used rather than crystal salt. Some manufacturers treat the potatoes with chemicals such as phosphoric acid, citric acid, hydrochloric acid, or calcium chloride to reduce the sugar level and improve the product's color.

What's in the Chip?

For starters, here's the nutritional information on the most popular potato chip on the planet.

> **Lay's Original:** 150 calories, 90 calories from fat: one gram of saturated fat, 4.5 grams of polyunsaturated fat, 4.5 grams of monounsaturated fat, 0 grams of trans fat, 0 grams of cholesterol, 180 milligrams of sodium, 330 milligrams of potassium, 1 gram of fiber, 0 grams of sugar, 15 grams of carbohydrates, 2 grams of protein

Lays has also made a low fat version, as follows:

> **Lay's Light Original:** 75 calories, 0 grams of fat, 0 milligrams of cholesterol, 200 milligrams of sodium, 17 grams of carbohydrates, 2 grams of protein

Lay's Light Original chips are slightly crunchier than their full-fat counterparts, and the extra 20 milligrams of sodium shows up as a slightly saltier tang. All together, these are a thoroughly satisfactory replacement for regular plain chips. However, like regular chips, they do leave a greasy mouth feel. For some, this is an attraction that drives them to pound down whole bags at a sitting.

> **Baked Lay's Original:** 120 calories, 2 grams of fat, 0 milligrams of cholesterol, 180 milligrams of sodium, 23 grams of carbohydrates, 2 grams of protein

These chips resemble "Pringles." And there's a reason for that: These chips are made from dehydrated potatoes, just like those famous canned chips. However, they are also somewhat doughier than Pringles, and I defy anyone to eat more than a few of them without running for a toothpick to remove vast quantities of starchy gunk from their gums. The flavor is adequate, but the soft crunch and mouth-clogging properties are unappealing.

> **Cape Cod 40 Percent Reduced Fat:** 130 calories, 6 grams of fat, 0 milligrams of cholesterol, 110 milligrams of sodium, 18 grams of carbohydrates, 2 grams of protein

The Cape Cod chips did very well in comparison. These are in every respect good chips. They don't have quite the crunch of the classic kettle-cooked chips, since a "flash baking" process is used, along with a dunk in the kettle to control the fat content, but they're still quite good. The one down-side had nothing to do with the crunch. The salt content seemed a bit lacking. A truly good chip has a salty kick, and that was oddly missing here.

Pringles Reduced Fat Original: 140 calories, 8 grams of fat, 0 grams of cholesterol, 135 milligrams of sodium, 17 grams of carbohydrates, 1 gram of protein

Just as with the Lay's Light Original, this was nearly impossible to tell apart from the original on which it was modeled. That addictive crunch was there, as well as that flavor, much like "Pringles." For fans of classic chips, these are not a great substitute, but if you prefer your chips in a can, these will make you happy.

Snyder's Soy Crisps Parmesan, Garlic and Olive Oil: 160 calories, 9 grams of fat, 0 milligrams of cholesterol, 290 milligrams of sodium, 11 grams of carbohydrates, 8 grams of protein

No, that sodium number is not a misprint. There are honestly 290 milligrams of sodium in each serving of these chips. What that serves to do is destroy the taste of the garlic or olive oil the bag claims to include. Essentially, if you were to open a can of cheap parmesan cheese in your refrigerator or cabinet and eat a heaping spoonful, it would resemble the flavor of these chips. The texture is more like a cracker than a chip but isn't bad. It has a blast of saltiness and lack of other flavors.

Doritos Light Nacho Cheese: 100 calories, 2 grams of fat, 0 milligrams of cholesterol, 200 milligram of sodium, 19 grams of carbohydrates, 2 grams of protein

The slightly spicy cheesiness makes Doritos one of the chip-aisle heroes. The crunch is a bit more cracker-like than the original chips, but still quite adequate. And, as a bonus, these chips don't turn your fingers orange quite as much as the originals. These are a tasty choice.

> **Flat Earth Garlic and Herb Veggie Chips:** 130 calories, 5 grams of fat, 0 milligrams of cholesterol, 190 milligrams of sodium, 19 grams of carbohydrate, 2 grams of protein

This name of this chip is a mouthful of words, and the flavor isn't bad either. It is slightly sweet, and the garlic flavor is most definitely present, in great contrast to the soy crisps. The texture isn't quite "chip," but isn't overly breaded. It is light and pleasing. This chip could be the next replacement to the overly greasy chip.

> **Ruffles Light Original:** 70 calories, 0 grams of fat, 0 grams of cholesterol, 190 milligrams of sodium, 17 grams of carbohydrates, 2 grams of protein

By now, it should come as no surprise that the fat-free chips taste very close to the originals, since they contain an indigestible fat substitute called Olestra or Olean. Fat substitutes offer the taste and feel of fats without any calories from fat. The chips overall are smaller than the usual Ruffles, but hold up just as well when dragged through the dip. Dip, of course, negates the "fat-free" qualities, but that's just the price you have to pay.

Side Effects of Olestra

Olestra is made by adding fatty acid chains to a molecule of sucrose (sugar). Our digestion can do nothing with it, and it is too large to move through the intestinal wall and be absorbed.

It creates two main consequences as it moves quickly through our digestive system. One consequence is that, since it is fatty in nature, it rapidly depletes blood levels of many valuable fat-soluble substances, including vitamins A, D, E, and K and carotenoids. The other consequence is that, since it is indigestible, it causes cramping and loose stools (diarrhea). The side effects are so common and so unpleasant that the FDA requires the following warning on all products that contain Olestra:

> "This Product Contains Olestra. Olestra may cause abdominal cramping and loose stools. Olestra inhibits the absorption of some vitamins and other nutrients. Vitamins A, D, E, and K have been added."

Although Olestra seems to be a great invention because it simulates what we like about fat, it creates an absolutely miserable experience for those who are sensitive to the side effects from it.

Snacking Between Meals

Between school, homework, sports, after work, and hanging out with friends, it may feel like there's no time for healthy eating. When you do stop to eat, it's probably tempting to go the quick and easy route by grabbing a burger and fries, potato chips, crackers or candy. But it is possible to treat yourself to a healthy snack. In fact, if you have a hectic schedule, it's even more important to eat healthy foods that give you the fuel you need to keep going. Even if you take time to eat three meals a day, you may still feel hungry at times. So what do you eat? How about a healthy snack? Snacking on nutritious food can keep your energy level high and your mind alert without taking up a lot of your time.

Why Healthy Snacking is Good for You?

You may have noticed that you feel hungry a lot if you're a teenager. This is a natural feeling during adolescence. A person's body demands more nutrients to grow. Snacks are a terrific way to satisfy that hunger and get all the vitamins and nutrients your body needs. But you need to pay attention to what you eat. Stuffing your face with a large order of fries may give you a temporary boost, but a snack this high in fat and calories will only slow you down in the long run. To keep energy levels going and avoid weight gain, steer clear of foods with lots of simple carbohydrates (sugars) like candy bars or soda. Look for foods that contain complex carbohydrates like whole-grain breads and cereals and combine them with protein-rich snacks such as peanut butter or low-fat yogurt or cheese.

Judging Whether Snacks are Healthy

Choosing healthy snacks means shopping smart. Be cautious of the health claims on food packages. Here are some things to watch out for. Just because something is "all natural" or "pure" doesn't necessarily mean that it's nutritious. For example, "all natural" juice drinks or sodas can be filled with sugar (which is, after all, a natural ingredient) but all that sugar means they'll be high in calories and give you little nutrition. A granola bar is a good example of a snack that people think is healthy for them. Although granola bars can be a good source of certain vitamins and nutrients, many also contain a great deal of fat, including trans fats. On average, about 35% of the calories in a regular granola bar come from fat. And there can be a lot of sugar in granola cereals and bars. Check the Nutrition Facts label on the package to be sure. Be skeptical of low-fat food claims, too. If the fat has been eliminated or cut back, the amount of sugar in the food may have been increased to keep the food tasting good. Many low-fat foods have nearly as many calories as their full-fat versions.

Whatever claims a food manufacturer writes on the front of the package, you can judge whether a food is healthy for you by reading the ingredients and the nutrition information on the food label.

Smart Snacking Strategies

Here are some ways to make healthy snacking part of your every day routine. Prepare your healthy snacks in advance. When you make something yourself, you get to control the ingredients and put in what's good for you! You can also keep plenty of fresh fruit and veggies at home so you can grab them on the go. Cut up melons or some vegetables like celery and carrots in advance. Keep the servings in bags in the fridge, ready to grab and go. Here are some additional ideas:

- Keep healthy snacks with you.
- Make your snacks interesting.
- Satisfy cravings with healthier approaches.
- Read serving size information.

As with everything, moderation is the key to smart snacking. People who eat regular meals and healthy snacks are less likely to overeat and gain weight than people who skip meals or go for long periods without eating and then scarf down a large order of fries. It's natural to feel hungrier at certain times, like during a long afternoon of classes or work. Knowing how much food your body needs to satisfy this hunger is very critical. A handful of walnuts make great brain food before sitting down to do homework or focus on business decisions. But a whole bag won't help you add anything except pounds!

Sport Snacks May Lack Nutritional Value

In all grocery stores, health food stores, sporting good stores, and convenience stores you go to, there are snacks. They are called energy bars, protein bars, power bars or cereal bars. They are conveniently packaged in individual servings for on-the-go eaters. Variably marketed as breakfast foods, meal replacements, dieters' supplements, or power boosters for athletes, the bars seek to fill different nutritional niches. Some offer high carbohydrates, some high protein, some a balance of both. No matter the nutritional angle, they all send comforting messages of good, clean living. And American consumers have responded with enthusiasm. But depending on the bars they choose, they could be undermining their dietary goals.

According to an article in Consumer Reports magazine, the nation spends a little over one billion dollars per year on brands including: PowerBar, Clif, Clif Luna, Carb Solutions, Atkins Advantage and Ultra-Slim Fast. "They're the Egg McMuffin for the health set," says Chris Rosenbloom, Associate Dean of Georgia State University's College of Health and Human Sciences. "They're something you can eat with one hand: in the car, on the cellphone, et cetera." "What it's all about is convenience," said Dianne Busenbark, a member of the technical sales staff at Phidippides, an Atlanta running equipment store that has been selling energy bars since they first hit the market in the late 1980s. "Runners don't have to pack a bagel or take a banana and let it get squished in their fanny pack. They pay for their PowerBar, and then they're on their way." Marlene Thomas, a running enthusiast who lives in Marietta, Georgia, can relate. She always keeps PowerBars within reach. "I carry them in the car, they're in my running bag, they're in the kitchen, they're everywhere," she said. "If I get hungry, I just open up a PowerBar. It's better for you than fast food."

Originally marketed as a carbohydrate boost for runners and other serious athletes, the product's nutritional mission has become muddled as its popularity has spread to other consumer groups. "It used to be, the people who were buying these things were the ones who were out every day for an hour or two," Busenbark said. "But now it's like a snack that's enjoyed by far more casual athletes," she observed. "They know they're working out, they feel like, 'I'm doing something, I deserve something.' But the problem with that reasoning, nutrition experts say, is that most people do not need the extra calories offered in so-called energy bars. And bars marketed as meal replacements may not provide the same quality of nutrition, or hunger satisfaction, as real food. To a nutritionist, energy just means calories. "If they called them calorie bars, no one would buy them," said Rosenbloom, a longtime nutrition consultant for Georgia Tech and Georgia State athletes. "For people trying to lose weight who are going to the gym or aerobics a few times a week, I'd stay away from all of these energy bars. They're probably going to sabotage your efforts." "Many of the brands marketed as meals on the run — called cereal, nutritional or breakfast bars are high in sugar and low in fiber," noted Rosenbloom. "A lot of these are basically candy bars," she said. "They may be fortified with vitamins and minerals, but they may be similar as far as fat and calorie content." Information printed on the packages for Special K breakfast bars indicates they are virtually identical, nutritionally speaking, to packaged Rice Krispies Treats; both are low in fat, but high in sugar and offer little in terms of vitamins and minerals. A gram-for-gram comparison between Quaker Chewy Trail Mix bars and 3 Musketeers candy bars suggests that although the Quaker bar has slightly more protein and significantly less sugar, the two have very similar caloric, total carbohydrate and fat contents.

Still, if the choice is between grabbing a fortified snack bar on the go or skipping breakfast, only to buy a candy bar two hours later, then the snack bar is a far better choice, said Mollie Katzen, a nationally known advocate of healthy eating and author of the new breakfast cookbook Mollie Katzen's Sunlight Café. "You go from feeling like having nothing to eat to feeling like eating the walls," she said of the classic breakfast skipper. "Going from those blood sugar swings is really not that healthy," said Katzen. Over the years, Katzen's dietary philosophy has evolved from a high-carbohydrate, low fat diet to a more balanced mix of protein, complex carbohydrates and high-quality unsaturated and non-trans fats. So, when shopping for healthy snacks for her family, she considers total calories, fiber content and protein content. She also tries to avoid all trans fats.

Here's a quick rundown of some of the nutritional benefits offered in ingredients that can easily be incorporated into healthy snacks:

- Dried fruit: iron potassium and selenium
- Protein antioxidants High in fiber: Nuts and nut butters
- Flax seed: Fiber omega-3 fatty acids
- Whole grains and whole-grain flours: Fiber, B vitamins, Vitamin E, Magnesium, Selenium and Zinc
- Wheat bran and wheat germ: High-fiber, high-nutrient portions of the wheat
- Honey: a natural ingredient with organic options; it's sweeter than more processed granulated sugar and therefore you typically need to use less if it

Conclusions

So, what have you learned? Well, not all alternative chips are necessarily gourmet delights, and it's possible to eat bad food with good intentions.

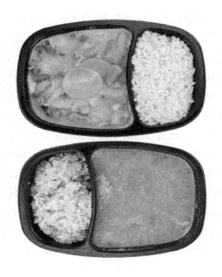

CHAPTER 8
FROZEN FOODS

History of Frozen Foods

Clarence Birdseye processed the first system for quick-freezing foods. This involved a key innovation, packing the food before freezing it. This simple idea had two main advantages. It reduced the food to convenient rectangular form, allowing direct contact with the freezing surface, and insulated it from the processing equipment, eliminating the sanitary problems of food touching processing equipment or chemicals. An advantage of freezing is that peas and other foods can be harvested and packed at their peak flavor, regardless of market demand at the time. Frozen-food companies employ field agents to keep close watch on crops, monitor their growth, and decide when they should be harvested. Harvested fruits and vegetables can usually be brought to a freezing plant in less than six hours.

Commercial packers use two basic methods of freezing. One of them is the convection method, in which packaged food moves along a conveyor belt while cold air is blown over it at about ten miles per hour. This method is used for irregularly shaped objects, such as whole poultry, and when it is desirable to keep items loose, as with peas in bags. In some cases, to save space, the conveyor is a stacked helix that carries the packages along a spiral path. The other method is Clarence Birdseye's conduction process, with metal plates containing refrigerant. This technique is more energy efficient and especially suitable for food packed in straight-sided boxes. The packages are loaded onto stacks of the plates and are slightly compressed while refrigerant runs through the plates. The temperature in each box is brought down to 25°F in a few minutes. Many kinds of refrigerant have been used, including brine, dichlorodifluoromethane (CCl_2F_2, also known as Freon-12) and various glycols. Now packers are switching to new refrigerants to reduce environmental damage, especially ozone depletion.

Is Frozen Food Safe?

Food stored constantly at 0°F will always be safe. Only the quality suffers with lengthy freezer storage. Freezing keeps food safe by slowing the movement of molecules, causing microbes to enter a dormant stage. Freezing preserves food for extended periods because it prevents the growth of microorganisms that cause both food spoilage and food borne illness. The freezing process itself does not destroy nutrients. In meat and poultry products, there is little change in nutrient value during freezer storage.

Enzymes

Enzyme activity can lead to the deterioration of food quality. Enzymes present in animals, vegetables and fruit promote chemical reactions, such as ripening. Freezing only slows the enzyme activity that takes place in foods. It does not halt these reactions which continue after harvesting. Enzyme activity does not harm frozen meats or fish and is neutralized by the acids in frozen fruits. Most vegetables freeze well, are low in acid, and require only a brief partial cooking to prevent deterioration.

Freezer Burn

Freezer burns do not make food unsafe, merely dry in spots. It appears as grayish-brown leathery spots and is caused by air reaching the surface of the food. Cut freezer-burned portions away either before or after cooking the food. Heavily freezer-burned foods may have to be discarded for quality reasons.

Refreezing

If you thaw food in the refrigerator, it is still safe to refreeze it without cooking, although there may be a loss of quality due to the moisture lost through defrosting. After cooking raw foods which were previously frozen, it is safe to freeze the cooked foods. If previously cooked foods are thawed in the refrigerator, you may refreeze the unused portion.

Look for the USDA or State Mark of Inspection

The inspection mark on the packaging tells you the product was prepared in a USDA or state-inspected plant under controlled conditions. Follow the package directions for thawing, reheating, and storing.

Daily Servings of Fruits and Vegetables

Americans typically eat only one-third of the recommended daily intake (three servings instead of nine) of fruits and vegetables, so if you're in a bind a vegetable in any form is better than no vegetable at all. As winter approaches, fresh produce is limited, expensive, or fresh only in distant parts of the country. This forces many of us to turn to canned or frozen options. Canned vegetables tend to lose a lot of nutrients during the preservation process (notable exceptions include tomatoes and pumpkin).

"Frozen vegetables may be even more healthful than some of the fresh produce sold in supermarkets," says Gene Lester, Ph.D., a plant physiologist at the USDA Agricultural Research Center in Weslaco, Texas. Fruits and vegetables chosen for freezing tend to be processed at their peak ripeness, a time when, as a general rule, they are most nutrient-packed. On the other hand, fruits and vegetables destined to be shipped to the produce aisles around the country are picked before they are ripe, which gives them less time to develop the full spectrum of vitamins and minerals. Outward signs of ripening may still occur, but these vegetables will never have the same nutritive value as if they had been allowed to fully ripen on the vine. In addition, during the long haul from farm to fork, fresh fruits and vegetables are exposed to lots of heat and light, which degrades some nutrients, especially delicate vitamins like C, the B vitamins and thiamin.

Bottom Line

When vegetables are in season, buy them fresh and ripe. "Off-season" frozen vegetables will give you a high concentration of nutrients. Choose packages marked with a USDA "U.S. Fancy" shield, which designates produce of the best size, shape and color. Vegetables of this standard also tend to be more nutrient-rich than the lower grades "U.S. No. 1" or "U.S. No. 2." Eat them soon after purchase. Over many months, nutrients in frozen vegetables do inevitably degrade. "Steaming or microwaving, rather than boiling produce will minimize the loss of water-soluble vitamins," says Rachael Moeller Gorman. "As freezing food is the most natural preservative in the world, it would be a waste of time to add anything."

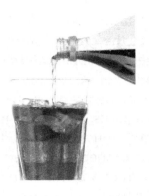

CHAPTER 9

JUICE AND SOFT DRINK AISLE

Juice is the extracted liquid from fruits or vegetables. These liquids can be a highly concentrated source of nutrition including vitamins, minerals, natural sugars, and healing phytonutrients. Juice is an easy way to add fruits and vegetables to any diet. But, the term juice can be used loosely. Many packaged, processed "juice drinks" or "fruit nectars" are loaded with artificial ingredients and sugar.

Varieties

Almost any fruit or vegetable can be juiced. Vegetable juices are lower in calories than fruit juices, and the most common are tomato, carrot and mixed vegetable juices. Fruit juices can be made from produce such as apples, pears, peaches, nectarines, apricots, prunes, cherries, berries, grapes, melons, citrus and tropical fruits.

Freshly squeezed or extracted juice made at a juice bar or in a home juicer has the best flavor. Fresh frozen juices are quickly frozen after extraction, without pasteurization, and retain most of the nutrients and taste. Chilled fresh juices, found in the refrigerated section of the grocery store, are freshly extracted juices that are packaged for shipping and distribution. Frozen juice concentrates are made from pasteurized juice from which the water has been extracted before freezing the solid, concentrated portion. Reconstituted juices, made from juice concentrates that have been pasteurized, must be labeled "from concentrates." One hundred percent canned or bottled juices may be made from a single fruit or from a blend of fruits to create a certain flavor and level of sweetness. Those made from a single fruit may be sweetened with grape juice. Like their frozen counterparts, canned concentrates made from evaporated pasteurized juices do not require refrigeration until they are reconstituted.

There are many fruit beverages or fruit drinks that contain only a small amount of real juice and may contain sugar, artificial flavors and colors. These drinks should not be counted as a fruit serving. Juice may be pasteurized or non-pasteurized. Pasteurization destroys many vitamins and minerals, but it also kills microbes and bacteria that cause spoilage and potential infection.

Buying and Storing Tips

All types of juice can be found in the grocery store. Look for fresh juices with pulp in the refrigerated section. Fresh-squeezed juice can be stored in the refrigerator for up to three days. Canned and bottled juices are usually found on store shelves and can be stored, unopened, in a cool, dark cupboard for up to three months. To preserve nutrient quality and taste, you should not store frozen juice and frozen concentrates in the freezer for more than one month. After opening, keep juices in tightly closed containers in the refrigerator. Pour servings and immediately refrigerate the closed container after every use.

Soft Drinks

From Wikipedia, the term soft drink (more commonly known as soda, pop, or soda pop in parts of the United States and Canada, or fizzy drinks in the U.K.) refers to carbonated drinks that do not contain alcohol. The name "soft drink" specifies a lack of alcohol in contrast to the term "hard drink." Beverages like colas, sparkling water, lemonade, and fruit punch are among the most common types of soft drinks, while hot chocolate, tea, coffee, milk, tap water, alcohol and milkshakes do not fall into this classification.

The History of Soft Drinks

Carbonated soft drinks trace their history back to the mineral waters found in natural springs. Ancient societies believed that bathing in natural springs and drinking mineral waters could cure many diseases. In the 1770s Joseph Priestley and other scientists made important progress in replicating natural mineral waters. Priestley infused distilled water with carbon dioxide. Another Englishman, John Mervin Nooth, improved Priestley's design and sold his apparatus for commercial use in pharmacies. Swedish chemist Torbern Bergman invented a generating apparatus that made carbonated water from chalk by the use of sulfuric fountains. Both men were successful and built large factories for fabricating fountain acid. Bergman's apparatus allowed imitation mineral water to be produced in large amounts. Soda fountain pioneers made artificial mineral waters, usually called "soda water." The soda fountain became an enormous moneymaker in the United States.

    Beginning in 1806, Yale chemistry professor Benjamin Silliman sold soda waters in New Haven, Connecticut. He used a Nooth apparatus to produce his waters. Businessmen in Philadelphia and New York City also began selling soda water in the early 1800s. In the 1830s, John Matthews of New York City and John Lippincott of Philadelphia began manufacturing soda.

The Origin of Cola

In the 1500s, the Spanish colonists noted how the Indians of South America were able to relieve fatigue by chewing the leaves of the coca shrub. However, that observation lay dormant for three centuries as the science of organic chemistry developed. This led to the extracton of the first pure crystals of cocaine from the coca leaf in small quantities. It was then used as a stimulant in beverages. By the 1880s in Paris, a druggist named Angelo Mariani created an immensely popular cocaine-laced wine (vin Mariani). It contained about 30 milligrams of cocaine in five ounces. Pope Leo XIII gave a gold metal to Mariani for being a benefactor of humanity.

In the late 1880s, in Atlanta, a new non-alcoholic drink was born to quench thirsts and provide pep during steamy summers. *Coca Cola* contained cocaine from the coca plant and lots of caffeine from the kola bean. Other ingredients were lots of sugar, caramel coloring, lime juice, citric acid, phosphoric acid, nutmeg, coriander, neroli (orange flavoring) and cinnamon. The new beverage was sold as syrup that would be mixed with cold soda water at local drugstores. In the 1930s a scoop of vanilla ice cream was added and it became a Coke float.

In 1906, congress passed Pure Food and Drug Act. The official in charge of its enforcement set out to prove that the 'Coca Cola habit' was harmful to health. By 1922, that official claimed in Good Housekeeping magazine that a child who drank three or four 6 ounce cokes a day would probably ruin his health for life. Today, we know why that's true.

Nutritional Value

Until the 1980s, soft drinks used refined cane sugar or corn syrup to obtain the soft drinks sugar contents. Today high-fructose corn syrup (HFCS) is used exclusively as a sweetener because of its lower cost. However, HFCS has been criticized as having a number of harmful effects on human health, such as promoting diabetes, hyperactivity, hypertension and a host of other problems. While the USDA recommended daily allowance (RDA) of added sugars is 10 teaspoons for a 2,000-calorie diet, many soft drinks contain more than this amount. Unless they are added, soft drinks contain little to no vitamins, minerals, fiber, protein, or other essential nutrients. Many soft drinks contain food additives such as food coloring, artificial flavoring, emulsifiers and preservatives. Some also argue that caffeine-containing soft drinks are not a valid source of dietary fluids because of the diuretic properties of caffeine.

Studies Showing a Correlation between Soft Drinks and Obesity

A study from Harvard shows that soft drinks may be responsible for the obesity in children in the United States over the last 20 years. From 1991 to 1995, adolescent boys in the U.S., on average, increased their daily intake of soft drinks from 345 milliliters to 570 milliliters. Dr. David Ludwig of the Boston Children's Hospital showed that school children drinking at least eight fluid ounces (240 milliliters) or more of regularly sweetened drinks daily will consume 835 calories more than those avoiding soft drinks. Children who drink soft drinks loaded with sugar tend to eat much more food than those who avoid soft drinks. Either those taking sugared drinks lack the same restraint on foods, or sugared drinks cause a rise in insulin that makes adolescents hungrier, causing them to eat more. Soft drinks (including diet soft drinks) are also typically consumed with other high-calorie foods such as fast food, (hamburgers and fries). Children who drink soft drinks regularly are fatter on average, in addition to being more likely to develop diabetes later in life. This finding is controversial, because children in much of the Third World also consume large numbers of soft drinks with even more sugar and do not share the same obesity rates as American children, suggesting that other factors are involved aside from sugar consumption in soft drinks. Suggested factors based on this study include physical activity and the fact that American soft drinks are sweetened with high fructose corn syrup instead of cane sugar.

In March 2006, the journal Pediatrics published a paper entitled "Effects of Decreasing Sugar-Sweetened Beverage Consumption on Body Weight in Adolescents: A Randomized, Controlled Pilot Study." The paper suggests that reducing consumption of sugar-sweetened beverages helps reduce body mass index in the heaviest teenagers. In contrast, drinking a single 12 ounce can of soda a day rendered more than 1lb of weight gain every month.

Soft Drinks Linked to Weight Gain and Type 2-Diabetes

In 2004, an eight-year study of 50,000 nurses showed a correlation that suggests drinking one or more sugar-sweetened beverages (such as soft drinks and fruit punches) per day increases one's risk of developing diabetes by 80% versus those who drink less than one such drink per month. This finding was independent of other lifestyle factors. It concludes, "Higher consumption of sugar-sweetened beverages is associated with a greater magnitude of weight gain and an increased risk for development of type-2 diabetes in women, possibly by providing excessive calories and large amounts of rapidly absorbable sugars."

Soft Drinks and Teeth

A large number of soft drinks are acidic and some may have a pH of 3.0 or even lower. Drinking acidic drinks over a long period of time can erode the tooth enamel. Drinking through a straw is often advised by dentists as the drink is then swallowed from the back of the mouth and does not come into contact with the teeth. It has also been suggested that brushing teeth right after drinking soft drinks should be avoided as this can result in additional erosion to the teeth due to the presence of acid.

Carcinogens (Benzene) in Soft Drinks

Benzene is a known carcinogen, or cancer-causing agent. Major soft drink companies have documented benzene contamination in soft drinks since at least 1990. It was originally thought that the contamination was caused by contaminated carbon dioxide, but research has shown that benzoates and ascorbic acid or erthorbic acid can react to form benzene.

In 2006, the United Kingdom Food Standards Agency published the results of its survey of benzene levels in soft drinks. In the study, 150 products were tested and four contained benzene levels above the World Health Organization (WHO) guidelines for drinking water. The agency asked for these to be removed from sale. The United States Food and Drug Administration released its own test results of several soft drinks and beverages containing benzoate and ascorbic or erythorbic acid. Five tested beverages contained benzene levels above the Environmental Protection Agency's recommended standard of five ppb. The Environmental Working Group has uncovered additional FDA test results which show the following results: of 24 samples of diet soda tested between 1995 and 2001 for the presence of benzene, 19 (79 %) had amounts of benzene in excess of the federal tap water standard of 5 ppb. Average benzene levels were 19 ppb, about four times the tap water standard. One sample contained 55 ppb of benzene, 11 fold over the tap water standards. Despite these findings, as of 2006, the FDA stated its belief that "the levels of benzene found in soft drinks and other beverages to date do not pose a safety concern for consumers."

How Healthy are the New Soft Drinks?

"The truth is that artificially sweetened soft drinks, even those fortified with vitamins and minerals are anything but natural and healthy," says Marion Nestle, New York University nutrition professor and author of *What to Eat*. "It is ridiculous to market soft drinks as healthy, but in today's marketplace consumers are demanding more healthy looking food, and beverages and soft drink manufacturers need to boost sales," she says. "Most consumers do not need the extra vitamins found in fortified soft drinks," she adds. "These beverages do not address the real health issues of our country of obesity, heart disease, or cancer," says Nestle.

University of Vermont researcher Rachel Johnson, PhD, RD, agrees. "It concerns me that we have so many ultra-fortified products where we virtually put a vitamin pill into a soft drink," she says. "The nutrients put into these soft drinks are not the shortfall nutrients that are lacking in our diets such as calcium, potassium, folate, or vitamin D." Johnson advises consumers to choose beverages that not only quench thirst but also deliver needed nutrients, such as 100% fruit juice.

Liquid Calories Add Up Quickly

"Lots of people don't think about what they are drinking and how it impacts the overall diet," says Johnson. "The average American gets 22% of their calories from beverages." Indeed, a recent study from Yale University analyzed 88 soda studies and found a clear link between soft drink intake and consumption of extra calories. "The most compelling studies showed that, on days when people drink soft drinks, they consumed more calories than on the days when they did not have soft drinks," stated study coauthor Marlene Schwartz of WebMD. "When you do want to drink a soda, think of it as dessert," Johnson suggests. "If we treated a can of regular soda like a dessert, it would help keep extra calories under control," she says.

Soft Drinks, Diet Drinks and Weight Gain

Another scientific study looked at seven to eight years of data on 1,550 Mexican-American and non-Hispanic white Americans aged 25 to 64. Of the 622 study participants who were of normal weight at the beginning of the study, about a third became overweight or obese.

For regular soft-drink drinkers, the risk of becoming overweight or obese was:

- 26% for up to 1/2 can each day
- 30.4% for 1/2 to one can each day
- 32.8% for 1 to 2 cans each day
- 7.2% for more than 2 cans each day

For diet soft-drink drinkers, the risk of becoming overweight or obese was:

- 36.5 for up to 1/2 can each day
- 36.5% for up to 1/2 can each day
- 37.5% for 1/2 to one can each day
- 54.5% for 1 to 2 cans each day
- 57.1% for more than 2 cans each day

For each can of diet soft drink consumed each day, a person's risk of obesity went up 41%.

There are Many Uses for a Can of Coke

- In many states (in the U.S.) the highway patrol carries two gallons of Coke in the truck to remove blood from the highway after a car accident.
- You can put a T-bone steak in a bowl of Coke and it will be gone in two days.
- To clean a toilet: Pour a can of *Coca-Cola* into the toilet bowl and let the "real thing" sit for one hour, then flush clean. The citric acid in Coke removes stains from vitreous china.
- To remove rust spots from chrome car bumpers: Rub the bumper with a crumpled-up piece of Reynolds Wrap aluminum foil dipped in *Coca-Cola*.
- To clean corrosion from car battery terminals: Pour a can of *Coca-Cola* over the terminals to bubble away the corrosion.
- To loosen a rusted bolt: Apply a cloth soaked in *Coca-Cola* to the rusted bolt for several minutes.
- To bake a moist ham: Empty a can of *Coca-Cola* into the baking pan, wrap the ham in aluminum foil, and

bake 30 minutes. Before the ham is finished, remove the foil, allowing the drippings to mix with the Coke for sumptuous brown gravy.
- To remove grease from clothes: Empty a can of coke into a load of greasy clothes, add detergent, and run through a regular cycle. The *Coca-Cola* will help loosen grease stains. It will also clean road haze from your windshield.
- The active ingredient in Coke is phosphoric acid. Its pH is 2.8. It will dissolve a nail in about 4 days.
- To carry *Coca-Cola* syrup (the concentrate) commercial trucks must use the 'Hazardous Material' placards reserved for highly corrosive materials.
- The distributors of Coke have been using it to clean the engines of their trucks for about 20 years!

Contents in Soft Drinks

Soft drinks usually contain the following components: phosphoric acid, caffeine, sugar, Spenda, aspartame or saccharin, caramel coloring, carbon dioxide and aluminum. Ingesting a soft drink does not cause an immediate warning symptom such as stomach cramps, vomiting or diarrhea that would normally occur when a poison enters the body. Instead, there is the energizing feeling from caffeine, the sweet taste of sugar combined with the sour taste of phosphoric acid, and the playful feeling of the carbon dioxide bubbles. These ingredients cause imbalances in body systems resulting in debilitating diseases that show up after many, many years of abuse. Those diseases have now become commonly thought of as normal aging with no directly attributable causes.

Phosphoric Acid

Phosphoric acid creates an acid medium that enhances the absorption of carbon dioxide (which also forms carbonic acid in water), thus reducing the pressure required for carbonation and allowing the mixture to be bottled with a metal cap. The carbon dioxide bubbles are released more slowly, particularly if the mixture is chilled. The sour taste of the phosphoric acid is complemented by adding lots of sugar.

The body maintains a concentration of phosphorus (P) times calcium (Ca) to equal potassium (K), or (P x Ca = K), in the bloodstream to provide the right combination for building new bones and remodeling old ones. The shock of incoming phosphorus with zero calcium in a soft drink causes ionized Ca in the blood to decline, along with an excretion of Ca in the urine. The drop in blood Ca causes another body system to dissolve Ca from the bones (taken from the teeth, spine and pelvic bones) to make up for the imbalance caused by the Ca lost in the blood. This process, continued over time, results in a weakened bone structure (osteoporosis) associated with older people. The body dissolves more Ca from the bones than is needed in anticipation of more phosphoric acid shocks. The excess of Ca has to be rerouted, generally in the following order depending on how much extra Ca has to be handled:

- Excretion in the urine
- Deposition in joints (causing osteoarthritis, bursitis, gout, bone spurs and bunions)
- Accretion into stones (kidney stones, etc.)
- Deposition in arteries (calcified plaque)

Phosphoric acid is the same material that cleans deposited materials in your shower. It is such a strong chemical that a tooth will dissolve in it. Phosphoric acid, like coffee, causes the body to use its alkaline minerals (sodium, potassium, magnesium, and calcium) to neutralize the acid. The body loses valuable minerals because the neutral compounds (salts) are excreted in the urine. Sodium depletion causes bile to become acidic and form mucoid plaque on the intestines, which causes colitis and other serious bowel diseases. Potassium and magnesium depletion can contribute to the development of heart disease. Phosphoric acid is physiologically such a strong acid that causes the body to reduce secretion of hydrochloric acid (HCl) used for digestion of protein and fats and absorption of minerals, leading to inadequate digestion resulting in bloating and gas. Poor absorption of dietary iron can result in anemia, and poor calcium absorption accelerates the trend of osteoporosis. Another not-so-obvious harmful effect of low stomach acidity is the overgrowth of harmful bacteria, yeasts and parasites in the gastrointestinal (GI) tract that had been held in check by adequate HCl. These creatures can break down the protective mucosal lining, penetrate into the bloodstream, lodge in organs and cause the formation of carcinogens that provoke cancer.

Caffeine

This chemical is an addictive drug that has the ability to stimulate mental alertness, overcome fatigue, and enhance endurance, but at a price. Caffeine acts by blocking adenosine (neurotransmitter) receptor sites in the central nervous system. Adenosine has a generally depressant action in the brain, heart and kidneys. These results can cause constriction of the cerebral arteries, rapid heartbeat, high blood pressure and excessive excretion of urine. Caffeine causes the release of adrenaline and an accompanying upshot in blood sugar to meet the need for emergency energy. The pancreas also reacts by secreting insulin to keep the blood sugar level stable. Insulin drives blood sugar levels down by forcing it into cells for oxidation and energy production. Excess sugar is stored as fat. This unbalanced cycling process puts undue stress on the adrenal glands and the pancreas, which are weakened after so much use. Adrenal exhaustion and the accompanying deficiency of cortisol allow arachidonic acid to be released to form prostaglandin-2 and leukotrienes which mediate arthritis. Regular users who are deprived of daily caffeine are subject to mental sluggishness, inability to think clearly, depression, and a dull, generalized headache. All these symptoms are promptly eliminated by caffeine. Even moderate users must have their daily fix and cannot give up their harmful habit.

Caffeine addiction is difficult to break because caffeine's penalty to health is not immediately recognized, and it is easy to deny. The addiction of caffeine, sugar and powerful advertising make the soft drink a superior method for the delivery of ingredients that taste great, but are unsuspectingly destructive to health.

Aspartame, Saccharin and Caramel Coloring

Aspartame is a sweetener that has found its way into almost everything, except baked goods, to replace sugar.

Saccharin is a sweetener that is also a carcinogen (causing cancer) in animals. In 1978, the National Academy of Sciences concluded that saccharin is a potential cancer-causing agent in humans, and that it promotes the carcinogenic effects of other agents. The Food and Drug Administration's position is that saccharin should not be used in food, but it is used as a table sweetener!

Caramel coloring is obtained by heating sugar until a brown color and characteristic flavor develops. Caramel coloring has negative genetic effects and can be a cancer-causing agent.

Aluminum

When it was found that phosphoric acid eats away enough aluminum from the inside of cans to be harmful, the problem was 'solved' by plastic-coating (Teflon) on the interior of the aluminum can. However, phosphoric acid still leaches toxic amounts of aluminum into the soft drink despite the plastic coating. Aluminum is deposited in the brain and bone tissue. Aluminum results in the formation of neurofibrillary tangles in brain tissue. The same type of lesions is seen in the brains of individuals who suffer from Alzheimer's disease. Aluminum exposure increases the amount of bone breakdown while at the same time reducing new bone formation. Aluminum causes excessive loss of calcium in the urine.

Parents are Top Influence on Soft Drink Consumption among Kids.

A Study in the *Journal of the American Dietetic Association* looked at trends in what kids drink and why flavored, carbonated drinks have been around for about two hundred years. And their popularity continues to grow, overtaking more nutritious beverages among some age groups, especially children and adolescents. Researchers at the University of Minnesota surveyed 560 children ages 8 to 13 years old on how often they drank soft drinks and the factors that influence their soft drink consumption. Among other findings, researchers found: Parental soft drink intake has a stronger influence on children. Parents who consume soft drinks on a regular basis may relax soft drink consumption rules and restrictions for their kids.

Approximately 30 percent of children reported drinking soft drinks daily and 85 percent reported they usually drink regular, not diet soft drinks. Soft drink consumption was higher among boys compared with girls and intake increased with age. Ninety-six percent of surveyed said that they like or strongly like the taste of soft drinks. Those children who reported that they "strongly like" the taste of soft drinks were 4.5 times more likely to drink soft drinks five or more times per week. The odds of drinking soft drinks almost daily was twice as likely for those who watched television 3.5 hours or more a day than those who watched less television. The availability of soft drinks at home and the availability of soft drink vending machines in school were both strongly associated with children's soft drink consumption.

The Bottom Line

The experts agree that there is no harm in enjoying a 'low' or 'no-calorie' soft drink occasionally. They also point out that the additives in some of the new sodas, no matter how healthy sounding, are either unnecessary or are added in such small quantities that they do nothing for improving your health. Consume the most natural foods and beverages, and always read the label. Check calories first, followed by sugar calories. Equipped with the facts, you can select the drink that's right for you. And keep in mind, that soft drinks have no place in diets. Soft drinks do not belong in the diet of young children. They need so many nutrients for growth and development, there is little room for soft drinks, and even then it should only be an occasional treat. American Dental Association (ADA) Spokesperson Althea Zanecosky says, "Parents need to be aware of what their kids are consuming and encourage foods and beverages that are packed with nutrients. As your best guideline, be sure soft drinks are not crowding out water and other nutritious beverages like unsweetened fruit juices."

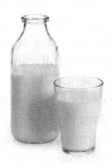

CHAPTER 10

DAIRY AND EGG DEPARTMENT

Milk

How wholesome is your milk? Industrial farms use a number of methods for increasing milk production in dairy cows, including selective breeding, feeding grain based diets (instead of grass) and exposing cows to longer periods of artificial light.

One of the most common and controversial ways to force greater milk production is to inject cows with rBGH (recombinant bovine growth hormone). This is the genetically engineered form of bovine growth hormone, developed and manufactured under the brand name Posalic, by Monsanto Corporation. rBGH has been a controversial issue from the start. rBGH is also referred to as rBST, or recombinant Bovine Somatotropin. The FDA approval for rBGH came in 1993, in spite of strong opposition from scientists, farmers and consumers. According to scientists, rBGH was never properly tested. The FDA relied solely on a study done by Monsanto in which rBGH was tested for 90 days on 30 rats. The study was never published, and the FDA stated the results showed no significant problems. But a review by the Canadian health agency on rBGH found the 90-day study showed a significant number of issues which should have triggered a full review by the FDA.

A 1991 report revealed serious health problems with the rBGH injected cows that were part of a Monsanto financed study at the University of Vermont. Among the problems was an alarming rise in the number of deformed calves and dramatic increases in mastitis, a painful bacterial infection of the udder which causes inflammation and swelling. To treat mastitis outbreaks, the dairy industry has relied on antibiotics. Critics of rBGH point to the increase in antibiotic use, inadequacies in the federal government testing (which contributes to the growing problem of antibiotic resistant bacteria), and antibiotic residues in milk as further reasons why the hormone should never have been approved. Additionally, cows forced to produce unnaturally high quantities of milk will often become malnourished because they lose more nutrients through their milk than they ingest in their feed, and are therefore more susceptible to disease.

By the summer of 1994, the Wisconsin Farmers Union and the National Farmers Union set up a joint hotline for dairy farmers to use when reporting problems with artificial growth hormones in cattle. One lifelong New York dairy farmer reported losing a quarter of his herd to severe mastitis after beginning the use of rBGH. Cows were suddenly producing less milk than they had before going on the drug. A year later, he had to replace 135 of his original 200 cows. Other farmers using rBGH have reported similar problems such as hoof diseases, open sores and cows that died from internal bleeding.

Scientists have linked the rise in twin births over the last 30 years to consumption of bovine growth hormone in the food supply. Milk from rBGH treated cows contains higher levels of IGF-1 (Insulin-like Growth Factor 1), which has been linked to colon and breast cancer. Even though no direct connection has been made between elevated IGF-1 levels in milk and cancer in humans, scientists have expressed concern. Faced with mounting evidence to the contrary, the FDA has stubbornly continued to assure consumers that rBGH is safe for cows and humans. In fact, in 1994, the FDA prohibited dairies from claiming there was any difference between milk from rBGH injected cows and milk produced without the hormone.

Did You Know?

According to Science News, 80 percent of all U.S. feedlot cattle are injected with hormones. A study of cows treated with melengestrol acetate (an artificial growth hormone approved for use in the U.S.) revealed that residues of this hormone were traceable in soil up to 195 days after being administered to the animals. While the average dairy cow produced almost 5,300 pounds of milk a year in 1950, today a typical cow produces more than 18,000 pounds.

Do Hormones Remain in the Milk or Meat of Treated Animals?

The levels of naturally produced hormones vary from animal to animal. Because it is not possible to differentiate between the hormones produced naturally by the animal and those used to treat the animal, it is difficult to determine exactly how much of the hormone used for treatment remains in the meat or the milk. Studies indicate that if correct treatment and slaughter procedures are followed, the levels of these hormones may be slightly higher in the treated animal's meat or milk, but still within the normal range of natural variation known to occur in untreated animals. Scientists are currently trying to develop better methods to measure steroid hormone residues left in edible meat from a treated animal.

Can Hormone Treated Cows Be Cause of Breast Cancer?

Once again, evidence does not exist to answer this question. Use of rBGH for dairy cattle has not been in practice in US for many years. Breast cancer can take many years to develop. It is too early to study the breast cancer risk of women who drink milk and eat milk products from hormone treated animals.

Concerned About Milk-Related Allergies?

A detailed discussion of this topic is beyond the scope of this fact sheet. A brief outline of the issue is presented here, along with references for more information. Digested or broken down fragments of proteins absorbed through the stomach can cause the immune system to produce antibodies which sometimes can lead to milk related allergies. There have been studies done to investigate whether the immune system can react to fragments of rBGH and IGF-1 absorbed through the stomach. Reviewers of these studies at Health Canada (the Canadian counterpart to the FDA) expressed a concern that in one study some of the laboratory rats that were fed high levels of rBGH for 90 days developed antibodies against it.

Scientists at the FDA evaluated these studies in rats and concluded that only animals that were fed a very large amount of rBGH in food produced antibodies against it. Such large amounts of rBGH are not expected to occur in the milk that humans drink ("Report on the Food and Drug Administration's see: *Review of the Safety of Bovine Somatotropin.*") Studies have also looked at whether IGF-1 fed to laboratory rats and digested in the stomach can affect the immune system. No immune effects were observed in these studies, but the animals were fed IGF-1 for only two weeks. No studies have been done on the effects of feeding rats or other experimental animals with IGF-1 over longer periods of time.

What about Growth Factors in Milk of Treated Animals?

The wholesomeness of milk is not affected by rBGH treatment. However, some changes do take place in the treated animal. The growth hormone usually acts by triggering the cells to make other chemicals, called growth factors. These growth factors actually cause the increase in growth rate and milk production.

Scientists at the FDA have considered the evidence from studies of cancer risk in people who have naturally high body levels of IGF-1. Higher levels of IGF-1 in blood have been found in women with breast cancer compared to women without breast cancer in the Harvard based Nurses' Health Study. Scientists are investigating if IGF-1 is just present at higher levels in breast cancer patients or if it has a role in increasing the risk for the disease. FDA scientists have concluded that IGF-1 in milk is unlikely to present any human food safety concern for the following reasons:

- IGF-1 levels in cow's milk from untreated animals vary in nature, depending on the number of calves and the lactation stage

- IGF-1 is also present in human breast milk, at levels higher than in hormone treated cow's milk

- IGF-1 in milk is not expected to act as a growth factor in people who drink it because it gets digested in the stomach

- IGF-1 needs to be injected into the blood to have a growth promoting effect

- IGF-1 increased levels in food are not expected to result in higher blood levels of in humans who eat the food

The Egg

Surrounded by the eggshell, the slimy, clear fluid of the egg is the albumen, egg white, the egg's cytoplasm. It consists of 90% water, seven major proteins, and no fat, according to the USDA's National Nutrient Database. Textbook descriptions of albumen note that ovalbumin is the main protein, making up 54% of the white.

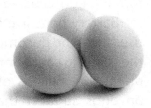

Yolks contain all of the vitamins in the egg, including six B vitamins, as well as vitamins A, D and E. The yolk also contains the antioxidants lutein and zeaxanthin and trace amounts of beta-carotene, phosphorus, iron, magnesium and other minerals.

Modern hens that lay eggs for human consumption are frustrated birds forced to live inside small wire cages. These chickens are classified as battery caged birds. Tiers of identical cages in sheds hold 50,000 to 125,000 birds. By nature an energetic scavenger, the hens should be ranging by day, perching at night, and enjoying cleansing dust baths with their flock mates.

Caged for life without exercise while constantly drained of calcium to form egg shells, battery hens develop the severe osteoporosis of intensive confinement known as caged layer fatigue. Calcium depleted, millions of hens become paralyzed and die of hunger and thirst inches from their food and water.

In the 20th century, the combined genetic, management, and chemical manipulations of the small Leghorn hen have produced a bird capable of laying an abnormal number of large eggs, up to 250 a year. This is in contrast to approximately 140 laid by her wild relatives. Battery hens suffer from the reproductive maladies that afflict female birds deprived of exercise. Masses and bits of eggs clog their oviducts which become inflamed. The battery cage has created an ugly new disease of laying hens called fatty liver hemorrhagic syndrome, characterized by an enlarged, fat, friable liver covered with blood clots. They also have pale combs and wattles covered with dandruff. In recent decades, hen oviducts have become infested with salmonella bacteria that enter the forming egg, causing food poisoning in consumers.

Battery hens live in a poisoned atmosphere. Toxic ammonia rises from the decomposing uric acid in the manure pits beneath the cages to cause ammonia-burned eyes and chronic respiratory disease in millions of hens. Studies of the effect of ammonia on eggs suggest that even at low concentrations significant quantities of ammonia can be absorbed into the egg. Hens to be used for another laying period are force-molted to reduce the accumulated fat in the reproductive systems and to regulate prices by forcing the hens to stop laying for a couple of months.

Battery hens are debeaked. Debeaking is done to offset the effects of the compulsive pecking that can afflict birds designed by nature to roam, scratch, and peck at the ground all day, not sit in their cages. To save feed costs and promote conversion of less food into more eggs, debeaked birds have impaired grasping ability and are in pain and distress, eating less, flinging their food less and "wasting" less energy than free-range birds.

The battery system depends on debeaking and antibiotics. Many of the antibiotics used to control the rampant viral and bacterial diseases of chickens in crowded confinement can also be used to manipulate egg production. For example, virginiamycin is said to increase feed conversion per egg laid, bacitracin to stimulate egg production, and oxytetracycline to improve eggshell quality. In factory farming virtually 100 percent of laying hens in the United States are routinely dosed with antibiotics.

To date, there are no federal welfare laws regulating poultry raising, transport or slaughter in the United States. There is no reason to assume the industry will reform of its own accord. In our present society, no one is working to improve the conditions under which chickens are raised, transported, and killed.

Plenty of chickens are raised completely free-range. This means they get to chase bugs, scratch for seeds and eat grass in the fresh air and sunshine. For the laying hens it means the eggs are hard-shelled and the yokes are almost orange. Free range eggs are a great source of omega-3 fatty acids, beta-carotene, and vitamin E with about half the cholesterol of factory-raised eggs. Free-range hens are not debeaked and aren't given growth hormones, antibiotics or chemicals of any kind.

What Can You Do?

There are many small family farmers who don't use artificial hormones on their animals. By purchasing your milk and meat from local, sustainable farms, you are supporting a system that ensures the health and welfare of the farm animals and protects you and your family from hormone related health risks. You can choose hormone free beef and rBGH free dairy products at supermarkets. Foods that carry the "USDA certified organic" label cannot contain any artificial hormones. When purchasing sustainable raised foods without the "organic" label, be sure to check with the farmer to ensure no additional hormones have been administered. Visit the Eat Well Guide for an online listing of stores, restaurants and producers that sell hormone free meat and dairy products.

Tips For Consumers

- Give your kids "natural" or certified organic meat when possible.
- Read labels to find out whether the meat is hormone-free.
- Most natural beef and poultry does not contain hormones or antibiotics.
- Organic animals are more strictly regulated. They can only be fed 100% organic feed

A "Certified Organic" label guarantees the consumer the farmer adheres to the regulations in the National Organic Program and has been certified by an independent agency. For sources of natural beef, see the Institute of Agriculture and Trade Policy's consumer guide on beef, *Eat Well, Eat Antibiotic free*. If you can't find organic meat near you, see: www.organicconsumers.org directory of organic companies. And, if you simply can't afford it, limit kids' intake of non-organic meat and substitute with more beans, fruits and vegetables. See the *New Green Diet* by Joan Gussow, Ed.D, for more information.

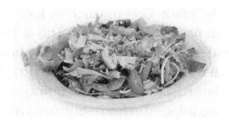

CHAPTER 11
CONCLUSION

Reasons to Choose Locally Grown Fruits and Vegetables

The health problems associated with modern diets are clearly worldwide in scope, and several national programs to raise public awareness are beginning to address these problems. However, there is an important missing element that may be waiting in our own backyards. There is considerable evidence that eating lots of fruits and vegetables is good protection against many diseases. What is not always as well recognized is the nutritional bonus of produce grown close to home. Locally grown fruits and vegetables have important advantages: nutrition, flavor, variety, economics and environment.

Flavor

Even though good nutrition is important, most people eat food for pleasure. It is the natural sugars and freshness that give freshly picked vegetables their tasty and delicious flavors. In many vegetables, such as sweet corn and peas, these natural sugars begin converting into bland tasting starch as soon as they are separated from the plant. Greens, such as kale and collards, are sweetest and most flavorful after a frost. This is because the plant protects leaf tissues from freezing by converting stored starch into soluble sugars. Another way flavors are lost from fruits and vegetables over time is from naturally occurring esters evaporating into the air. Produce shipped in from southern California or Mexico will never see a frost and much of their natural sugars and flavors are lost in storage on the long trip to your table.

Fresh Picked Vegetables are Sweeter

Introducing young children to fresh picked vegetables help them to enjoy fresh foods more and to develop the habit of eating that way the rest of their lives.

Increasingly, good restaurants and gourmet shops prefer locally grown produce when possible because the flavor is superior. This is a trend that creates significant markets for locally grown crops.

Nutrition

Ideally, crops should be harvested at the point in the plant's development when the level of nutrients is the highest. Immediately after harvest the nutritional value begins to fall. Produce shipped from distant farms has two distinct nutritional disadvantages when compared to local produce. First, it is likely to spend a longer time losing nutritional value between harvest and eating. Secondly, it is usually picked well before its peak of nutrition so that it won't wilt or spoil before it is sold.

Diversity

Many grocery stores carry a wider range of imported produce, such as mangoes and avocados. It is interesting, however, to remember the enormous diversity of locally grown fruits and vegetables that used to be available to us. One of the great things about local produce is that you can get varieties that are chosen for their taste and nutrition, not for how well they hold up to mechanical harvest and shipping.

Economics

One hundred years ago most states grew the food the local people ate. Now almost all states, including agricultural ones, get the bulk of their food from outside their boundaries at a high cost. As more of our produce started coming from huge mechanized farms thousands of miles away, the economy of many rural communities suffered.

Environment

It has been estimated that each bite of food in the U.S. has been hauled an average of 1,300 miles from the farm to the market shelf before being eaten. Transport of fruits and vegetables is especially demanding on the environment. Being comprised of about 85% water, most fruits and vegetables have a very short shelf life and quickly lose economic as well as nutritional value during shipping. Because of this, much of the produce that is hauled across the U.S. is delivered in refrigerated trucks that require even more fuel per mile than ordinary transport vehicles. To put this in perspective, consider every tractor-trailer load of produce that can be grown in the eastern U.S. instead of shipped in from southern California. Can you imagine how many gallons of fuel that wouldn't be needed for transportation?

In the heart of winter, we can produce lettuce and other cool-weather crops in simple greenhouses for a small fraction of the environmental cost of shipping them from southern California or Mexico. While we may well continue to haul in oranges and bananas from more tropical climates, it seems irresponsible to continue importing vast amounts of produce that could be easily grown closer to home.

Take Responsibility for Your Health

"Eat right and exercise," is the popular mantra we often hear. While it sounds easy, the problem is it's not that simple. Times have changed. How well is the public actually doing when they think they are eating right and exercising enough? Here are the unhealthy statistics on our American population: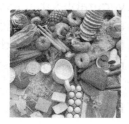

- 1 out of 2 will suffer heart disease
- 1 out of 3 will be diagnosed with cancer
- 1 out of 4 will develop diabetes, etc.

There were only 4 autoimmune diseases in 1970, now there are now over 80 new ones!

If it were easy to be healthy, EVERYONE would be healthy. Eating right is becoming more and more difficult as our soils are depleted, our air and waters are contaminated, and our plants are sprayed with toxins, harvested green, then preserved or gassed to ripen. We are seeing the results of this as our children suffer "adult diseases" earlier and more young couples are "infertile." Adults feel even more stressed and tired than ever before. Our immune systems are overtaxed, run down and incapable of coping.

Waxed and Pesticide Sprayed Fruits and Vegetables

When you bite into an apple or eat any other wax-coated produce, you could also be ingesting minute amounts of toxic chemicals. Washing the produce can get rid of almost all of these substances. All it takes is some diluted liquid dish soap and a sturdy vegetable brush. Of course, the more expensive soaps and other products sold specifically for cleaning produce work, too. After scrubbing, be sure to rinse well.

Another strategy is to peel off the skin when you can. For example, you can remove the skin from apples or cucumbers. Wax or no wax, pesticides still pose a problem. For non-waxed vegetables like lettuce, remove the outer leaves, which are likely most to be contaminated. Rinse the inner leaves before eating. Also consider buying organic produce, which typically has been exposed to fewer chemicals to begin with.

What about Exercise?

No one will argue exercise oxygenates our blood and gets our hearts pumping, but exercise without supplementation is also part of the problem. What we have long ignored is that when we exercise, we do not sweat out pure H_2O, but a soup of nutrients vital for our health and longevity. (That's why couch potatoes tend to live longer than Olympic athletes!) Exercise also increases our level of oxidative stress, producing free radicals that bombard our cells and DNA. Supplementation of depleted nutrients and antioxidants are necessary along with exercise.

If you are reading this, I believe it's because you recognize it's time you take responsibility for your own health! In today's changing environment, the pursuit of good health and longevity includes the "intelligent use of food supplements." This is a good investment for your own longevity.

What Food is Really Important?

Fruits and vegetables help not only in the digestive tract, but they also aid in cholesterol reduction and blood pressure regulation.

Primary foods that increase inflammation include coffee, soda pop, sugars and simple starches, flour, hydrogenated oils, trans fats, and red meats and dairy. Other sources of inflammation can be attributed to aspirin, acetaminophen and ibuprofen. We take these for pain and they actually inhibit the formation of cartilage.

Oils that help with inflammation are flaxseed and fish oils, both excellent sources of omega-3 essential fatty acids. These oils are considered the good oils. They build great cell membranes and bring down inflammation throughout the body. Other foods that contain omega-3s are extra virgin olive oil, coconut oil, shea nuts, ginger, even chia seeds. Good proteins give us amino acids to help assemble our building blocks to good nutrition. Proteins also help balance our blood sugar. Whey protein and tofu are both good meat alternatives. Other proteins are fish, eggs, chicken and turkey.

Read the Labels, and Fill Your Cart with the Most Nutritious Foods

It all starts in the grocery store. The foods you choose to stock your pantry, refrigerator and freezer are the foundation for your diet. Grocery shopping can be intimidating. It can be overwhelming to try to choose the healthiest foods from among all the options that line every aisle. New trends and choices pop up every day, from fortified foods to upscale gourmets.

To help you navigate the supermarket, here are some expert tips to help you read food labels and choose healthy products.

Label Reading Tips

The first thing you'll see is the label on the front of the food package. Manufacturers can say most anything they want on the front label. To get the real story, see the "Nutrition Facts" panel on the back.

Here are some terms you may see there, and what they really mean:

- Fortified, enriched, added, extra, and plus. This means nutrients such as minerals and fiber have been removed and vitamins have been added in processing. Look for 100% whole-wheat bread and high-fiber, low-sugar cereals.
- Fruit drink. This means there are probably little or no real fruit and lots of sugar. Look for products that say "100% Fruit Juice."
- Made with wheat, rye, or multigrain. These products may have very little whole grain. Look for the word "whole"

before the grain to ensure you're getting a 100% whole-grain product.

- Natural. The manufacturer started with a natural source, but once it's processed the food may not resemble anything natural. Look for "100% All Natural" and "No Preservatives."
- Organically grown, pesticide-free, or no artificial ingredients. Trust only labels that say "Certified Organically Grown."
- Sugar-free or fat-free. Don't assume the product is low-calorie. The manufacturer may have compensated by adding other ingredients for taste and this product may have no fewer calories than the real thing.

Key Phrases you will see on "The Nutrition Facts" Panel on the Back of the Package:

- Serving Size. Portion control is important for weight management, but don't expect manufacturers to make it easy for you. Pop-Tarts, for instance, come two to a package. The label says one serving is 200 calories - for "one pastry."
- Calories and Calories from Fat. This tells you how many calories are in a serving and how many of those calories come from fat. Remember that this information is for one serving as defined on the label.
- Nutrients by Weight and Percentage of Daily Value (%DV). This shows how much of each nutrient is in one serving, by weight in grams and by %DV. This symbol refers to the recommended daily allowance for a nutrient based on a 2,000-calorie diet (some nutrients, such as sugar and protein, don't have a %DV). Fats are listed as "Total Fat" and also broken down so you can see how much is unhealthy saturated fat and trans fats.

- Vitamins and Minerals. Vitamins and minerals are listed by %DV only. Pay particular attention to vitamin A, vitamin C, calcium and iron; most Americans don't get enough in their diets.
- Ingredients. These are listed in order from the greatest amount to the least. Experts offer a rule of thumb: the fewer the ingredients, the better.

Top 10 Foods to Put on Your Grocery List

Here are some foods that experts say should be on any health-conscious shopper's grocery list:

- Tomatoes. These juicy, red fruits are loaded with the antioxidant lycopene, which has been shown to reduce the risk of cardiovascular disease in women.
- Low-fat proteins. Good sources of lean protein include seafood, skinless white-meat poultry, eggs, lean beef (tenderloin, sirloin, eye of round), and skim or low-fat yogurts, milk and cheeses. Some research has indicated that a diet moderately high in protein can keep hunger at bay and help you lose weight.
- Whole grains, oats, and fibrous foods. Fiber helps your digestive tract work properly and lowers cholesterol levels while keeping your belly feeling full. Whole grains also contain antioxidants, are fat free, and are easy to fit into your diet.
- Berries (red and blue), including grapes. Berries are loaded with vitamins and minerals, as well as phytochemicals with cancer-fighting properties. Red grapes, in the form of one glass of red wine daily, may even reduce the risk of heart disease, according to the American Heart Association. Resveratrol supplements, (if you're a nondrinker) work much like drinking a glass of red wine a day.
- Nuts. A handful of almonds, cashews, pecans, or walnuts provides fiber, vitamin E, and healthful, monounsaturated

fats. Just watch your portion size; these nutritious nuggets are high in calories.

- Fish and fish oil contain omega-3 fatty acids that can reduce the risk of heart disease by protecting the heart against inflammation. The American Heart Association recommends eating fatty fish such as salmon, mackerel, tuna or sardines at least twice a week.
- Unsaturated fats such as olive, canola, and soybean oils are the best kind of fats.
- Low-fat dairy products provide plenty of calcium to help keep bones and teeth strong are a great source of protein and may even enhance weight loss, according to some research.
- Vegetables are a healthful eater's best friend. All veggies, except avocados, are fat-free and loaded with disease-fighting phytochemicals. Legumes (like pinto, garbanzo, kidney, black beans and lentils) are underrated for their real nutritional value. The lowly bean is naturally fat free and loaded with protein, fiber, vitamins, and minerals, especially iron. They add few calories, but keep you feeling full.

Supermarket Savvy

This checklist offers healthier food choices in every department of your supermarket:

- Fruits and Vegetable. Spend the most time in the produce section, the first area you encounter in most grocery stores (and usually the largest). Choose a rainbow of colorful fruits and vegetables. The colors reflect the different vitamins and other nutrients. They are most economical when they are in season. If not in season, canned, frozen vegetables and fruits are a good way to consume minerals, and phytonutrients. Compare cost of fresh, frozen, and canned vegetables and fruits on a ready-to-serve basis. Get to know the desirable characteristics of fresh fruits and vegetables. Example: An orange or grapefruit that is heavy for its size is the best buy. Buy only those vegetables and fruits that look fresh and are free of wilt, bruise and decay.

- Breads, Cereals, and Pasta. Choose the least processed foods that are made from whole grains. For example, regular oatmeal is preferable to instant oatmeal. But even instant oatmeal is a whole grain, and a good choice. When choosing whole-grain cereals, aim for at least four grams of fiber per serving. The less sugar, the better. Keep in mind that one level teaspoon of sugar equals four grams and let this guide your selections. Avoid granolas, even the low-fat variety; they tend to have more fat and sugar than other cereals.

- Bread, pasta, rice, and grains offer more opportunities to work whole grains into your diet. Choose whole-wheat bread and pastas, brown rice, grain mixes, quinoa, bulgur and barley. To help your family get used to whole grains, you can start out with whole-wheat blends and slowly transition to 100% whole-wheat pasta and breads.

- Meat, Fish, and Poultry. The American Heart Association recommends two servings of fish a week. Salmon is recommended because people often like it and it and it is widely available, affordable, not too fishy, and a good source of omega-3 fatty acids. Be sure to choose lean cuts of meat (like round, top sirloin, and tenderloin), opt for skinless poultry, and watch your portion sizes.

- Dairy. Dairy foods are an excellent source of bone-building calcium and vitamin D. There are plenty of low-fat and nonfat options to help you get three servings a day, including drinkable and single-serve tube yogurts, and pre-portioned cheeses. If you enjoy higher-fat cheeses, no problem- just keep your portions small.

- Frozen Foods. Frozen fruits and vegetables (without sauce) are a convenient way to help fill in the produce gap, especially in winter. Some of frozen foods include whole-grain waffles for snacks or meals, portion-controlled bagels, 100% juices for marinades and beverages, and plain cheese pizza that you can jazz up with an extra dose of skim mozzarella cheese and a variety of veggies.
- Canned and Dried Foods. Keep a variety of canned vegetables, fruits, and beans on hand to toss into soups, salads, pastas or rice dishes. Whenever possible, choose vegetables without added salt, and fruit packed in juice. Tuna packed in water, low-fat soups, nut butters, olive and canola oils, and assorted vinegars should be in every healthy pantry.
- DO NOT buy cans that are badly dented (especially on the seams) or that are bulging on the ends. The food in such cans may be spoiled and dangerous to eat.
- Select fruit juices that are high in vitamin C and other nutrients. Soft drinks and many canned and bottled fruit drinks and punches may have little or no vitamin C and will provide empty calories in the form of sugar.

Get The Facts. "%Daily Values"

The amount of nutrients in food is stated two ways: in grams (or milligrams) or as a percentage of the "Daily Value."

The "Daily Value" shows how a serving of food fits in with current recommendations for a healthful daily diet. These reference numbers called "Daily Values" are based on the government's Dietary Guidelines; for example, one guideline recommends restricting fat intake to 30 percent or less of calorie intake.

The government has set 2,000 calories a day as for calculating the "Daily Value." Of course, not everyone eats this amount. Teen-age girls often average 2,200 calories a day, while some teen-age

THE GROCERY STORE MYTH

boys may eat 2,500 or more calories a day. Whatever your calorie intake, you still can use the "Daily Values" on the label to get a general idea of how a serving of food fits into the total daily diet.

The goal is to eat about 100 percent of the "Daily Value" for each nutrient each day. For nutrients that may be related to health problems—such as fat, saturated fat and sodium, the lower the percent the better the choice. For other nutrients that are often needed to maintain good health and which may be in short supply—such as fiber and calcium--the goal is to eat at least 100 percent.

A good rule of thumb is this: if the "Daily Value" listed on the panel is five or less, the food contributes a small amount of that nutrient to the diet.

Enjoy your food and enjoy your life. Remember,

"Happiness is feeling good all over."

REFERENCES

2000 Healtheon /WebMD. All rights reserved.

Sylvia Davis WebMD
Weight Loss Clinic - Feature

Review by Louise Chang, MD

For additional information read *"10 Tips for Healthy Grocery Shopping. "*Published February, 2006.

SOURCES: Kathleen Zelman, MPH, RD. WebMD feature *"How to Read a Nutrition Label,"* by Leanna Skarnulis, published Aug. 13, 2004.

©2006 WebMD Inc. All rights reserved.

Introduction: Information by Jan Castagnar

Dietary Guidelines for Americans 2005. Center for Nutrition Policy and Promotion, U.S. Department of Agriculture.

Hung HC, Joshipura KJ, Jiang R, et al. *Fruit and vegetable intake and risk of major chronic disease.* J Natl Cancer Inst 2004; 96:1577–84.

Appel LJ, Moore TJ, Obarzanek E, et al. *A clinical trial of the effects of dietary patterns on blood pressure.* DASH Collaborative Research Group. N Engl J Med 1997; 336:1117–24.

Djousse L, Arnett DK, Coon H, Province MA, Moore LL, Ellison RC. *Fruit and vegetable consumption and LDL cholesterol*: the National Heart, Lung, and Blood Institute Family Heart Study. Am J Clin Nutr 2004; 79:213–7.

Vainio H, Bianchini F. IARC *"Handbooks of Cancer Prevention: Fruit and Vegetables." Vol. 8. Lyon, France, 2003.*

Giovannucci E, Ascherio A, Rimm EB, Stampfer MJ, Colditz GA, Willett WC. *Intake of carotenoids and retinol in relation to risk of prostate cancer.* J Natl Cancer Inst 1995; 87:1767–76.

Gann PH, Ma J, Giovannucci E, et al. *Lower prostate cancer risk in men with elevated plasma lycopene levels: results of a prospective analysis.* Cancer Res 1999; 59:1225–30.

Giovannucci E, Rimm EB, Liu Y, Stampfer MJ, Willett WC. *A prospective study of tomato products, lycopene, and prostate cancer risk.* J Natl Cancer Inst 2002; 94:391–8.

Etminan M, Takkouche B, Caamano-Isorna F. *The role of tomato products and lycopene in the prevention of prostate cancer*: a meta-analysis of observational studies. Cancer Epidemiol Biomarkers Prev 2004; 13:340–5.

Lembo A, Camilleri M. Chronic constipation. N Engl J Med 2003; 349:1360–8.

Aldoori WH, Giovannucci EL, Rockett HR, Sampson L, Rimm EB, Willett WC. *A prospective study of dietary fiber types and symptomatic diverticular disease in men.* J Nutr 1998; 128: 714–9.

REFERENCES

Brown L, Rimm EB, Seddon JM, et al. *A prospective study of carotenoid intake and risk of cataract extraction in US men.* Am J Clin Nutr 1999; 70:517-24.

Moeller SM, Taylor A, Tucker KL, et al. *Overall adherence to the dietary guidelines for americans is associated with reduced prevalence of early age-related nuclear lens opacities in women.* J Nutr 2004; 134:1812-9.

Cho E, Seddon JM, Rosner B, Willett WC, Hankinson SE. *Prospective study of intake of fruits, vegetables, vitamins, and carotenoids and risk of age-related maculopathy.* Archives of Ophthalmology 2004; 122:883-92.

Krinsky NI, Landrum JT, Bone RA. *Biologic mechanisms of the protective role of lutein and zeaxanthin in the eye.* Annu Rev Nutr 2003; 23:171-201.

Harvard School of Public Health

From: *NewsTarget.com*
Source: *www.newstarget.com/007024.html*

Sunday, May 01, 2005

By Mike Adams

Baker , BP. *"Pesticide residues in conventional, integrated pest management (IPM)-grown and organic foods."* Nutrition Action July 2007:

DeCarlo, Tessa. *"The Better Beef Guide."* Organic Style (2004): 1–5.

Palmer, Sharon. *"Organic Beef."* Today's Dietitian 9(2006): 36–42.

Roosevelt, Margot. *"The Grass-Fed Revolution."* Time (2006): 1–4.

"The National Organic Program." USDA National Organic Program Standards. 2007. United States Department Of Agriculture. 16 Jul 2007

http://www.ams.usda.gov/nop/NOP/NOPhome.html

Learn more about drug resistance from the *"World Health Organization."*

Copyright © 2006 Scout News LLC. All rights reserved

Source: Ag and Resource Policy Report, Colorado State University

Randy Dotinga, Health Day Reporter

Posted: 13 October 2006 04:14 pm ET (Health Day News)

Bonnie S. BenwickWashington Post Staff Writer Wednesday, February 23, 2005; Page F01

Garret Leiva, Herald Editor Written by Gloria Tsang R.D., Published in January 2006 Written October 20, 2004

Deborah Geering: Cox News Service

Deborah Geering writes for The *"Atlanta Journal-Constitution."*

5 Ways to Lose Belly Fat: Stop making these 5 major mistakes & you'll finally lose the belly fat:*www.BellyFatIsUgly.com*

Carbohydrates Enjoy healthy dining with these free low carbohydrate recipes.*www.dLife.com*

REFERENCES

Good Carbs Bad Carbs Get 1000 tasty, healthy, right-carb recipes with Custom Online_Plan: *www.SouthBeachDiet.com* The *"high glycemic carbs"* are to be avoided and the *"low glycemic carbs"* are to eaten more often.

Reviewed by: Mary L. Gavin, MD
Date reviewed: March 2006
Originally reviewed by: Jessica Donze Black, RD, CDE, MPH

Author,Jan Castagnar

Author, Samantha Broaddrick

(Source: Heaney RP, Rafferty K. *Carbonated beverages and urinary calcium excretion.* American Journal of Clinical Nutrition 2001,74:;343–347

http://www.hc-sc.gc.ca/english/archives/rbst). *"The Use of Steroid Hormones for Growth Promotion in Food-producing Animals Brief,"* overview of hormones used in food animals. (Center for Veterinary Medicine, U.S. Food and Drug Administration, July 2002)

Utah State University Beef Cattle Implants. An explanation of the process used to implant hormones into beef cattle, and a list of the various hormones commercially available. Although the authors state hormone-treated meat is safe for human consumption, they do not explain how they determined its safety. (Utah State University, August 2000)

Potential Public Health Impacts Of The Use Of Recombinant. Bovine Somatotropin In Dairy Production. This paper begins to assess the safety of the use of rBGH (recombinant bovine growth hormones), and discusses the issue of IGF-1 (Insulin Growth

Factor I). (Prepared for a Scientific Review by the Joint Expert Committee on Food Additives, Consumers Union. Janet Raloff, *Science News Online,* January 2002)

EU Scientists Confirm Health Risks of Growth Hormones in Meat. An *Associated Press.*

Article reports that a European Union scientific panel has confirmed eating beef from cattle raised on growth hormones is a potential health risk. *Associated Press,* April 23, 2002 Sources

This page is dedicated to my friend Dr. Joe Brown, NMD. I admire his commitment and courage helping people understand how they can battle, conquer and overcome the obstacles of cancer.

Cancer Survivor Now Cancer Doctor

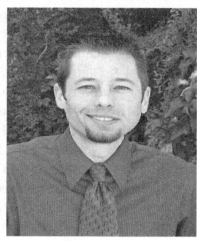

Dr. Joe Brown - Naturopathic Doctor,

-Winner of the Spirit Award- 2008-Presented by Channel 3 T.V.-Good Morning Arizona

-CoHost of 1310 Independent Radio

-Winner of the Hero Award- 2008 from 104.7 F.M.-Radio Station, Phoenix Arizona

-Featured in the INCURABLES Series, Satellite & Cable T.V. (Cancer Survivor, Now Cancer Doctor!) www.DrJoeBrown.com

Dr. Joe Brown, Naturopathic Physician, offers more to his patients than knowledge and expertise. He offers his personal experience in battling cancer. In 1998, Dr. Brown was diagnosed with late stage III melanoma cancer. After going through extensive therapy he was told his prognosis was grim. Through the use of Naturopathic and Integrative Medicine, he was able to overcome that prognosis. His cancer has been in remission for over 10 years.

Dr. Brown's passion stems from his personal experience in battling cancer and being told his only two options for survival included chemotherapy and radiation. He has focused on learning all he can about new and innovative therapies that have been shown to be successful in treating cancer. Through his expertise in Integrative Oncology, Immunology, and his personal battle,

Dr. Brown helps patients diagnosed with cancer through their journey. It is important to him to supply the missing pieces that will support the conventional therapies of chemotherapy and radiation; bridging conventional medicine and natural therapies, creating a better prognosis.

His quest and passion to make a difference in others lives led him to open his own clinic, Natural Health Medical Centers, in which all patients even those who are being treated with chemotherapy and/or radiation therapy can begin other treatments such as I.V. Therapy, Iscador injections, Injection Therapy, Acupuncture, Nutritional & Diet changes, and supplementation. Using these therapies simultaneously aids elimination of side effects of traditional treatments and stimulates the body's innate immunity so chemotherapy and radiotherapy can be most effective. Thus, utilizing both worlds of care, Dr. Brown provides the patient the absolute best treatment from both schools of thought.

Dr. Brown is an active member of the Arizona Association of Naturopathic Physicians (AANP), Naturopathic Public Awareness Campaign (NPAC) and the Oncology Association of Naturopathic Physicians (OncANP). He has spoken at numerous Open House events at Southwest College of Naturopathic Medicine and at Arizona State University. His lectures include dendritic T-cell stimulation, life style choices that lead to cancer, stimulation of the immune system, and his own personal battle with cancer and how he beat it.

Phone: (602)-421-2613
CancerAlternatives@DrJoeBrown.com
www.DrJoeBrown.com

Family Medicine, Acupuncture, IV Therapy, Chronic Pain, Nutritional Counseling, Fatigue, Heart Disease

---

Natural Health Medical Centers
2055 E. Southern Avenue, Suite B, Tempe, Arizona 85282

Notes

Notes

Notes

Notes.

Made in the USA
Middletown, DE
30 October 2024

63020159R00096